The
Holistic
Gardener

Natural Cures for
Common Ailments

The
Holistic
Gardener

Natural Cures for
Common Ailments

Fiann Ó Nualláin
Illustrations by Sam Chelton

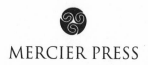

MERCIER PRESS

DISCLAIMER: This book is a collection of skills and advice compiled by a gardening expert. This book should not be used as a medical guide in the purest sense: the author is not a trained doctor, although the contents are reliable and could be useful for the ailments described. Before using the remedies the reader must ensure all plants mentioned are correctly identified and processed as described. If serious illness is suspected medical help should be sought immediately. The publisher can accept no responsibility for any consequences of advice given here or any illness caused in the practice of the techniques or remedies described, nor of any prosecution relating to the treatment of people which may adhere directly or indirectly to the techniques or remedies described in this book. The reader should assume full responsibility for any practical use of any of the techniques and remedies described. If in doubt, consult a medical practitioner or qualified herbalist.

MERCIER PRESS
Cork
www.mercierpress.ie

First published in hardback in 2016. This edition first published in 2018.

© Text: Fiann Ó Nualláin, 2016

© Illustrations: Sam Chelton, 2016 (excluding pages 44, 51, 115, 141)

ISBN: 978 1 78117 623 8

10 9 8 7 6 5 4

A CIP record for this title is available from the British Library

Printed and bound in the EU.

For my mam, Bernadette, who first taught me the power of a dock leaf over a nettle sting, vinegar over an insect sting, a lick of spit over a scratch and a bar of chocolate over a bruised knee.

CONTENTS

INDEXES

INTRODUCTION

This is the third book in the *Holistic Gardener* series of books – each one aimed at promoting an engagement with the functionality or 'full potential' of what we can easily grow in our backyard or front garden – exploring how we can harvest our gardens and allotments for natural treatments and better health. The two previous books – *First Aid from the Garden* and *Beauty Treatments from the Garden* – both hit bestseller lists and received much praise. Each book had a tight focus: the first was tailored for 'first aid' needs, the second for specific 'beauty' issues. However, with the topic 'common ailments' the spectrum is much broader. In order to provide well-researched answers to the individual complaints, I have narrowed the list to 1) ailments that are commonly occurring; 2) ailments that make up the majority of visits to the GP or trips to the chemist; 3) ailments that are not conditions – they are 'illness events' rather than a long-term illnesses; 4) ailments in which natural treatments can have an impact, be that as a supplement to conventional medical treatments, or as an alternative to over-the-counter medications.

This book, like the rest of the *Holistic Gardener* series, is about a self-empowered, self-sufficient approach to health. I am a gardener and a herbalist; I witness every day how nature heals and empowers. Self-sufficiency is not frugality. It is more than ecological consciousness. It is taking control. It is engaging resilience and acquired abilities (the skills of growing, home crafting and even straightforward cooking) to direct energies into your personal welfare and well-being. Some of the ailments discussed in this book are transitory; some can be debilitating. So whether you're involved in a skirmish or a full-on battle, I hope this book gives you the weapons and strategies you require to win. Being fighting fit is a good thing and many of the entries, especially in the 'Kitchen support' sections, aim to treat the ailment by getting you to optimum health.

When I was young I loved martial arts – as much for the honourable and spiritual pathways as for the physical and mental challenges – and from that time and those experiences I still carry valuable life lessons and strategies. One was to aim *behind* the target, not at the target – to punch through, not slow your punch to land. So the herbs and foods I choose to treat the ailments don't just land a blow, they travel through, have further impact. They not only treat the complaint, but also boost your immune-system response, get your neuroreceptors reacting, kick-start your energy centres, or detox your system. That's fighting fit. That's the knockout punch.

Before I end up as 'the Kung Fu Gardener' I should just say that, in terms of my holistic gardener credentials, I have spent much of my life studying and exploring horticulture, medicinal botany, ethnobotany (the personal and cultural uses of plants within anthropologies), healing modalities, complementary medicine and holistic practices. So don't be surprised when you find the answer to your ailment may be an acupressure point, a yoga move or a meditation technique – or a berry from a shrub and not just a herbal tea: it's whatever works best for the situation. Of course, I do include herbalism, nutritional therapy, aromatherapy and so on where relevant.

As a gardener by profession and passion, this book is written with gardeners in mind. But the natural way is for everyone, so there are no plants that are troublesome to grow and no techniques that require prolonged expertise to master. There are no fret factors here: health is hard enough to attain and retain without that. So enjoy the book, enjoy your garden and enjoy health.

GLOSSARY

Adaptogenic – helps the body cope with stress

Analgesic – relieves pain

Antiemetic – prevents vomiting

Antihistamine – counteracts histamine

Antioxidant – improves blood flow and immune response

Antispasmodic – eases the spasm reflex

Antitussive – suppresses coughs

Anxiolytic – reduces anxiety

Bacteriostatic – stops bacteria from multiplying

Carminative – speeds up digestion and reduces gas

Demulcent – soothing

Diaphoretic – promotes perspiration

Diuretic – promotes the production of urine

Emmenagogue – triggers blood flow in the uterus

Expectorant – helps to loosen and expel mucus

Febrifuge – reduces temperature

Hepatic protective – strengthens and detoxifies the liver

Lymphagogue – promotes the flow of lymph

Mucilage – a soothing, gelatinous substance

Nervine – soothes the nerves

Styptic – causes bleeding to stop

Vasodilating – widens the blood vessels

THE NATURAL APPROACH

Herbalism is not a fad, *food as medicine* is not an ancient pre-Tweet – they are strategies for health from our earliest ancestors to our current generations. Plants and foodstuffs have always been used for medicinal purposes – long before recorded history their use was captured in folklore and ethnobotany, and, in many cases, detailed at the dawn of the move from oral to written traditions. Ancient Chinese scrolls and Egyptian papyri detail medicinal uses for plants and food as early as 3000 BC, and that knowledge, combined with indigenous practices from across the world, influenced western medical practices and the development of modern medicine.

So how did we lose herbalism as a mainstream practice? The industrial revolution and the capitalist/consumer system brought many changes – some good advances but some cul de sacs too. When chemical analysis first became available in the early nineteenth century many of the popular plant-based medicines were studied for commercial potential and industrial manufacture, and this meant extracting and modifying the active constituents from plants into chemical compounds. 'Standardisation' and 'convenience' pushed the pill over the potion and so herbalism went into decline. That said, it is estimated that almost a quarter of modern pharmaceutical drugs are derived from botanical sources. Today there is a keen interest in returning to those original sources as we deal with chemical sensitivities and an overload of commercial product. Many of us yearn for the natural. But does it work?

The answer is yes, and we know this because that's where modern pharma continues to get its inspiration and seek its patents. We know it works because modern science is reinvestigating the old cures, and papers and studies are giving validation on an ongoing basis. What we have forgotten is that in many cases it actually works better. This is often down to something we herbalists call 'plant synergy' – basically the herb (plant part) is more than one extracted phytochemical and includes a whole range of ingredients that heal. So while the drug version might switch off pain receptors as the plant part did – as with aspirin (acetylsalicylic acid/$C_9H_8O_4$) and the sources from which it was first synthesised, i.e. meadowsweet and willow bark (salicylic acid/$C_7H_6O_3$) – the other phytocomponents for allied support are missing from the synthesised versions. Both meadowsweet and willow bark, apart from being analgesic, have wider applications. Meadowsweet can be utilised for stomach complaints. Aspirin is not recommended for stomach complaints as salicylic acid and its derivatives are said to have the potential to cause internal bleeding from the stomach wall. So why does meadowsweet – loaded with salicylic acid – not need the same extreme caution? Well, in essence, because it is not just one constituent. The plant parts used also have polyphenols, which naturally protect the stomach lining. That's the synergy – there is a lot more going on.

One of the scaremongering mantras about natural medicines is that this 'lot more going on' can't be quantified in a lab – or has not yet been quantified in a lab. My answer is that herbalism, and holistic treatments in general, are as much about wellness as illness – the methods and modalities won't simply chemically kill 99 per cent of the bacteria causing the problem, they will also boost your own immune-system response to get you back to 100 per cent fitness, and also make your body better prepared for next time, if a recurring ailment is on your health radar.

Sometimes the 'more going on' is known as 'photosensitivity' – the herb may cause you to burn more quickly in the sun or to develop a rash that worsens on exposure to sunlight. Yet parabens and ingredients such as 6-Acetoxy-2 and 4-dimethyl-m-dioxane, which act as preservatives in sunscreen and some body lotions, are known photosensitisers. St John's wort (currently prescription only) and some other good herbs have been branded with causing photosensitivity – I am not denying that potential but I am also aware that parsnips, parsley, dill, fennel, celery and lettuce can all trigger photosensitivity. If you are prone to photosensitivity then St John's wort or parsley may be best avoided. I just find it intriguing that some medicinal herbs get a health warning that doesn't appear on common foods with the same risk factor.

The natural approach is a personal choice; I am not saying abandon all conventional medicine or stop taking your medications. I am simply suggesting that you can avail of the wonderful healing potential of your garden to remedy the ailments described in this book as you see fit. When you do, you can do it with the confidence that these herbs were the basis of the development of medicine – this is simply a return to the natural and one less chemical in your system today.

A WORD OF WARNING

Herbalism and home-crafted treatments are not necessarily suitable for every situation. Just as severe burns need medical attention and not a rub of aloe vera, certain skin conditions require the expertise of a dermatologist and particular pains are red flags for the attention of a medical professional. Also, not every remedy in this book will be appropriate for everybody. For example, people with an allergy to ragwort or other *Asteraceae* plants should of course avoid herbs in that family, and nut allergy sufferers should not make the flapjack recipe – yet for others they may be perfect choices. The seeds of hawthorn berries are stomach irritants and toxic in large doses but the fruit is edible and medicinal, while liver-detox herbs could strip prescription medications from your system before they get a chance to treat the relevant condition. Understanding the plants and the parts you harvest for use is vital when adopting a natural approach to recovery and sustained health. Choosing a natural approach is not a lesser option – in many instances it delivers better results and boosts overall health – but you need to strike a balance, find what works for you and what *your* best options are. So, while I will mention relevant facts, I also advise you to explore further or consult a herbalist to match your personal health history to the information in this book. The word of warning, as promised, is *judiciousness*!

INGREDIENTS AND CURRENT HEALTH STATUS

These remedies are based upon traditional treatments and ones I utilise or share with friends, but they do not, or more to the point cannot, take into account individual sensitivities and plant allergies, underlying conditions, current prescription medications that may interact and so on. So for all conditions, if you are unsure of the herb or your tolerance, consultation with a qualified herbalist or naturopath is recommended. Otherwise all the usual rules apply – caution with pregnancy, blood pressure, long-term-illness regimes and so on.

INGREDIENTS AND ETHICAL CHOICES

Some supplements mentioned in this book come from parts of the world where harvest exploitation could exist, but just as you may choose a Fairtrade coffee, your local health store can help you find an ecologically conscious and ethical brand. Where creams and lotions call for emulsifying wax, its inclusion is vital to make the oil and water contents mix. Emulsifying waxes can be either vegetable based or petroleum based. As the latter are by-products of crude oil, some home crafters and ecological gardeners may have reservations about them, so be sure to ascertain which type you require before purchase.

WORKING WITH HOME REMEDIES

Making home remedies is not only simple, it's also enjoyable. So fear not: this section gives you an insight into the process of home crafting a medicinal treatment.

Every ailment listed in this book has one or two dedicated recipes to address it – many laid out like cookbook recipes – which are simple to execute. All you need to do is follow the steps. No Bunsen burners or expensive knives are required. Some recipes are practically instant, as simple as tea to drink or a leaf blitzed in a blender with some vodka and rubbed in. Some may take a few weeks' infusing in oil or another base before being whipped up into a cream or lotion – but while the time required is long, the process is not time-consuming. Others are culinary in nature and, even though 'medicinal', they are tasty and formulated to easily fit into your lunch or as part of dinner in the evening. This is practical herbalism, so it must also be accessible.

In the 'Garden treatments' section of the various ailments I often discuss the possibility of including other herbs or methods to help the complaint. Or I simply list herbs that are antihistamine, analgesic and so on – you might wish to translate them into, say, a lotion or a tea. You can easily amend any of the lotions, potions, salves, creams, teas or rubs to incorporate these other herbs. All we are doing is extracting the phytochemical from the plant so that we can ingest it or absorb it through the skin. I will usually specify whether something is to be used internally or externally, or I may say, as a method, 'make a tea' (generally to consume) but clarify at certain times that it is for topical application or use as a rinse.

To help you explore more herbal treatment options, what follows is a brief guide to the basic extraction methods.

EXTRACTION METHODS

To make our treatments, we first need to obtain the phytochemicals from the plants. There are four main ways to do this.

WATER EXTRACTION

Many healing phytochemicals will quickly leach out of a plant into hot water (e.g. herbal teas and leaf infusions), while some will need to be decocted or boiled out (e.g. roots and twigs). Others can be retrieved by the hydrosol method. Hydrosols are also referred to as floral waters and are extracts produced by steaming plant materials. They are often considered 'aromatic waters' and can be used in aromatherapy, but because they retain the essential oils of the plant parts they have medicinal potential too.

How to make a basic hot-water infusion herbal tea

In general, 1 tablespoon of herbage to 1 cup (250ml) of hot water is the ratio required. Extra herbage can be added for a stronger extraction. Simply boil a kettle, pour the boiled water over the plant parts and steep for 5–10 minutes. Sometimes extra steeping is necessary for a specific treatment and this is noted in individual recipes.

How to make a basic decoction

Decoctions can be made from roots, bark, berries or foliage. Generally, 1–2½ tablespoons of herb per cup of water utilised will deliver a good decoction. In a saucepan (avoid aluminium saucepans if possible) bring the ingredients to a boil and then simmer for 20 minutes. Strain and cool. Only the strained liquid is used. Decoctions can be sweetened with a little brown sugar, molasses or honey to make a syrup. Decoctions and syrups can be refrigerated. Most decoctions will keep for three days, and syrups will keep for several weeks.

Decoctions can also be made by boiling plant parts in cider vinegar, beer or other liquids. A good tip is to crush, mash or score the plant parts just before boiling to extract the maximum amount of beneficial ingredients. Foliage easily releases its oils and other constituents into boiled water and so makes good tea and infusions, but roots and twigs often need to be boiled for quite a while. Many of the root and branch treatments in this book are decoctions.

How to make a hydrosol by steeping

Harvest some flowers and place the petals in a saucepan. Add just enough distilled or spring water to cover them, or no more than double the volume of the petals. Bring to a simmer. Cover and steep until the petals lose their colour and it leaches into the water. Strain and decant into a container. Hydrosols can be kept in dark glass bottles for several weeks if stored out of direct sunlight – ideally in a cupboard or other cool, dark location. You can extend the shelf-life to many months by adding 2 per cent high-proof vodka to the volume you have. Hydrosols can also be refrigerated for several weeks to a couple of months.

How to make a hydrosol by distillation

This method creates a pure essence similar to the witch hazel extract you can get from your pharmacy. Its concentration is stronger than that created by the steeping method. The process is more involved but it's worth it. First, make your makeshift still: you'll need a large pot, a slightly smaller lid, a cup, a small bowl and a tallish glass. Invert the cup in the centre of the pot. Then add petals to the pot and enough water to cover them, or no more than double the volume. Balance the bowl on top of the cup and place the tall glass in the bowl. Place the lid on top of the glass. The steam will hit the lid and form condensation, which will drip down the side of the glass into the gathering bowl. Bring the water to a simmer and keep it steaming, without allowing it to boil hard, for long enough to gather a decent amount of distilled essence. When the petals lose their colour, you can stop distilling. If balancing lids, bowls, cups and glasses gives you a panicky feeling, you can use cling film as a lid (weighted down with a stone in the centre). It will funnel the drips into the gathering bowl.

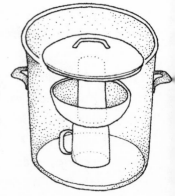

ACIDIC EXTRACTION

Other phytochemicals may need an acid to extract them. For this, you should use a safe acid such as vinegar or lemon juice. You can add herbs to your kitchen vinegar and infuse for a few days to a few weeks to make topical spritzes or medicinal washes. By adding vinegar or citric acid from fruit juice to the mortar and pestle mash, or when blitzing, you can obtain more constituents from the crushed plant parts.

How to make medicated vinegar

Empty the contents of a bottle of vinegar into a jug. Put as much herbage as will fit into the bottle and then refill with the reserved vinegar. Allow to sit for two weeks and then use as required. There's no need to strain off the solids – they may continue to leach phytochemical and aromatic ingredients for several more weeks, intensifying the treatment.

ALCOHOL EXTRACTION

Some of the most common over-the-counter herbal treatments are tinctures. First a simple solution is made by extracting plant elements into an alcohol base. The resulting liquid is often referred to as a mother tincture. This can be diluted and taken orally, or used neat as a topical rub or as an ingredient in other recipes. A tincture is as much a dosage as it is a preparation and usually consists of 10–20 drops of a mother tincture diluted in a glass of mineral water, three times daily for five days. Take a few days' break before beginning a second round of treatment.

How to make a mother tincture

The traditional way to make a tincture is using the menstruum method. It involves soaking half a cup of herbage in 2 cups (500ml) of vodka or brandy for four to five weeks. I prefer to use vodka, as the more noticeable colour change acts as an indication of complete extraction.

A quicker method is to blitz the same ingredients in a blender. Then pour into jars, place on a sunny window ledge and shake daily for a week. Allow to stand for a second week and then strain off the solids and bottle up.

OIL EXTRACTION

If an ingredient is fat-soluble – e.g. vitamin D – then an oil or a fatty substance is called for to help it leach out. Infused oils extend the seasonality (availability and storage) of the medicinal plants too.

How to make infused oil (sun method)

Simply fill a jam jar with as many plant parts (foliage, roots or petals) as will fit, cover completely with olive oil or any culinary oil you may have and place in a sunny window for a minimum of one to two weeks. This will allow the phytoconstituents of the herb to naturally leach into the oil.

How to make infused oil by heating

Using a bain-marie (a bowl suspended over a saucepan of boiling water), heat the oil (olive, almond, sunflower, etc.) and add your herbs. After 5–10 minutes, turn off the heat and allow the oil to rest and slowly infuse for a day or until it has fully cooled and is safe to work with. The beneficial constituents will continue to leach into the hot oil as it cools. For a more intense oil, you can simply fill a jam jar with herbs and oil, boil up some water and sit the jar in the water for an hour or so every day for several days to draw out as much goodness as possible. This is a cheat's version of the sun-infused oil.

In many cases the method of extraction is dictated by the intended use. For example, a thyme tea is a great antiseptic rinse to treat a cut or wound, but a thyme salve (thyme infused in an oil base and then set with beeswax) is great for healing and sealing moisture into chapped lips or hands. Similarly, using a different base can make an ingredient suitable for different applications. For example, calendula oil (the petals infused in some olive oil) can be used as a culinary aid to obtain fat-soluble vitamins A and D from foods in order to treat a deficiency-connected ailment. Or it can be set with beeswax, vegetable or nut butter to make a soothing skin cream. Herbs have a lot of versatility.

MEASUREMENTS AND METHODOLOGY

Most of the remedy recipes in this book are based on ratios, so as long as you're using the same cup or same size tablespoon, no technical difficulties should arise. We may be whipping up a lotion but we're not making soufflés! Even the food recipes are not complex. A margin for error is built in so a heaped teaspoon over a level teaspoon won't spoil the batch. You can scale up to mugs and even buckets if you wish, but small fresh batches are best. The cup measurement used in these recipes is equivalent to 250ml.

There may be subtle differences in thickness or texture if you use a store-bought dried herb over a freshly harvested garden-grown herb, but the phytochemicals and benefits of the plant are contained in both. This book is about easy engagement with nature and natural health, so a sprig of rosemary in a cup of vinegar or a handful of leaves in a footbath will often do the trick without turning your kitchen into a lab.

Where a degree of precision is necessary to achieve the proportions to effectively deliver the treatment, or to create a lotion and not a puddle, or a lozenge and not a toffee, I give specific measurements. In the remedy methods I give ratios or quantities that will yield an amount of product roughly equivalent to what you would normally buy.

If you keep your salve in a warm handbag or backpack as

opposed to a cool drawer or bathroom cabinet, it may be runnier some days and suitably set other days. Similarly if you stick with unadulterated emulsifying wax or raw shea butter, the outcome will be different than if you add emulsifying cream or a processed shea product. Variations are not a bad thing. The recipes contain no preservatives other than natural essential oils, alcohol and so on, so remember that shelf-lives are not infinite, which is no bad thing either.

And while this is all about handy treatments that are easily made and don't require a laboratory or any industrial processes, you should nevertheless consider preparation hygiene and sterile storage containers. The treatments are natural but they are still going on your skin or into your bloodstream, so avoid contaminating their natural goodness. Glass jars can be easily sterilised by putting them through the hottest dishwasher cycle or by thoroughly washing in soapy water, rinsing clean and then oven drying for 20 minutes at 120°C/gas mark 1.

STANDARDISATION AND DOSAGE

Standardisation is not easily achieved in home preparations. Seasonal variations apply and even a plant's growing aspect can be significant. Mint plants grown in full sun may have more aromatic oils than those in partial shade and so have more flavour and healing potential. Don't fret if your garden is not south facing – if a plant grows happily in your garden then it is producing the phytochemicals inherent in it and of benefit to us. Standardisation is not a factor in attaining those phytochemicals in either the quantities required or for the duration of use for the type of ailments in this book. We are making quick-fix cures, not treatments for life – the aim here is not management of a health condition, but relief and treatment of an ailment. We are not dealing with life-threatening, long-term or chronic conditions, but ailments that may arise from time to time and ones where, in many incidences, over-the-counter and prescription pharma treatments are based upon original plant cures. We are simply returning to the plant version.

As these are ailments – generally short-term conditions – it is not envisaged that you will use treatments or herbal supplements for a prolonged period. While all are safe, long-term self-medication of a complaint is not advised as it could mask a more serious underlying issue. If the ailment is prolonged or the cure is not healing with speed and efficacy, then you may need to look again at what is really going on.

A NOTE ON THE CONSISTENCY AND STORAGE OF HOMEMADE PRODUCTS

The recipes are not carbon copies of over-the-counter products or prescription medications. Where possible I have endeavoured to create a result close to what you can buy, but without the inclusion of chemical thickeners, preservatives and other agents that have no health value, the viscosity or texture of the cream or lotion may in some instances not match that of a conventional product, and sedimentation or separation can occur much sooner than with the commercial equivalent. You can shake the product before using or whisk again, but by making small batches, treatment timetables of several days to several weeks will be possible. The satisfying aspect of these remedies is how well they work as treatments.

Most of the remedies store well in airtight containers or are recommended for storage in the fridge, and their shelf-life expectancy is detailed. They are tailored to deal with specific, short-term ailments and are suited to short-term storage and usage.

THE AILMENTS

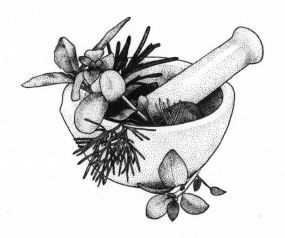

ACHES AND PAINS

Many visits to the local pharmacy are to find remedies for sundry aches and pains. These are also perhaps the most common complaints for gardeners due to the physicality of maintaining a garden and the potential for repetitive strain or just plain old injury – never mind the headache of greenfly. Whatever the source or intensity, help is at hand. Yet it is good to understand that pain is your body's way of saying something is wrong. If you know that it was just the incorrect lifting technique from earlier today or the way the hammer just hit that thumb, then, OK, reach for some natural 'aspirin' from the garden. If you are unsure why you have stomach cramps or severe pain anywhere in the body, then a visit to the GP is timely. I will explore the best options for specific pains under the relevant sections (see neuralgia on page 208, sprains and strains on page 198, backache on page 48, headaches on page 149), but here is some general advice that covers pain sensation.

Garden treatments

The garden can produce many herbal analgesics (pain sensation suppressants). Some are best taken as herbal teas, while others make great rubs or topical treatments. My favourite pain-relieving tea is fennel seed – the seeds are magic bullets packed with at least sixteen analgesic and twenty-seven antispasmodic phytochemicals, all yielding up into a cup of boiling water. Liquorice root is also excellent, with as many as ten analgesic and twenty anti-inflammatory phytochemicals, and you can't beat meadowsweet tea, hot or chilled. Meadowsweet was the inspiration for aspirin – in fact the word 'aspirin' takes its middle letters from meadowsweet's old botanical name *Spiraea Ulmaria* – and its similar compounds shut down pain receptors in a comparable manner to the drug.

Feverfew, as the name suggests, lowers fevers, but it also decreases the frequency and intensity of migraines and other headaches. Borage, evening primrose and blackcurrants are potent sources of pain-dampening gamma-linolenic acid (see more below). Daylily flowers are edible and a tea of the petals is slightly sedative and somewhat analgesic – it is used for pain relief in the ethnobotany of its indigenous growing regions. Topically, arnica – long lauded for shrinking bruises – with its phytochemical compound *helenin* delivers analgesic and anti-inflammatory results. Wintergreen is found even in over-the-counter creams for muscle and backache.

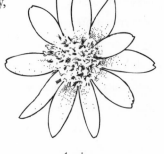

Arnica

Kitchen support

Coconut oil is analgesic both topically and internally (don't go swilling it; just a little will suffice in a curry or other culinary affair). Cayenne pepper and chillies contain capsaicin, which has a marvellous ability to naturally dampen pain perception, but its heat also triggers the release of pain-relieving endorphins. It is great in dietary terms and also in rubs, liniments, salves and massage-oil blends. Stem ginger or ginger root in cuisine or infusion (both oil and herbal tea) is analgesic and anti-inflammatory. Turmeric powder or root contains a compound known as curcumin, which has anti-inflammatory properties comparable to cortisone. It similarly acts upon pain receptors to lessen their communication potential – especially the neurotransmitter substance P that signals pain. Many of the common culinary herbs – thyme, rosemary, basil and oregano – have analgesic, antispasmodic and anti-inflammatory compounds. Even ordinary tea (black or green) is subtly relaxing and dulls pain perception.

If you are in prolonged pain then you might consider increasing your intake of gamma-linolenic acid (GLA), an omega-6 fatty acid which has a role in repairing nerve damage and works to decrease inflammation and pain perception. You can obtain it from blackcurrants, hemp seeds, spirulina and other dietary sources. GLA encourages the production of leukotrienes, prostaglandins and other hormone-like substances that stimulate and support the immune system. This helps to target underlying triggers of pain and plays a role in neutralising toxic accumulations in the system. A couple of weeks should show a remedial difference, but it can take four to six months to fully kick in.

Pain-relief Cuppa

Camellia sinensis, which is the source of green and black tea, contains nine muscle-relaxing compounds, while the tops of meadowsweet are packed with pain-suppressing salicylic acid.

Method

Depending on how strong you like your tea, add a teaspoon or tablespoon each of tea leaves and chopped meadowsweet to a pint of boiling water. Steep for a minimum of 5 minutes before straining. Honey and lemon are OK to flavour it with, but sip without milk or sugar. This is delicious as iced tea too.

ACID REFLUX AKA GASTROESOPHAGEAL REFLUX DISEASE (GERD)

Acid reflux is a condition where the acidic gastric juices of the stomach (sometimes accompanying regurgitation of food) rise into the oesophagus – irritating the lining as well as sections of digestive tract en route – resulting in burning sensations in the throat and often in the chest known as heartburn (see page 167). Heartburn is not always present and sometimes the reflux happens at night, unbeknownst to you or 'silently', but ancillary symptoms include difficulty swallowing during the day or the sensation of a lump in your throat upon waking, prolonged sore throat with hoarseness, stomach discomfort and occasionally sinus problems (see page 219).

The causes of acid reflux or GERD can include an inefficiency of the lower oesophageal sphincter to close off, or abnormal oesophageal contractions – often a symptom of stress (see page -237). Sometimes a hiatal hernia is implicated, or a case of slowed digestion (the stomach not emptying quickly enough) with excess digestive enzymes and gastric juices forming to counter the full stomach (see digestive complications on page 99).

Garden treatments

Several garden herbs, including rosemary, chamomile, catnip, lemon balm, basil and peppermint, are utilised for their soothing effects on the stomach and digestive system, and also for their ability to reduce the spasms that enable reflux. Fennel seed tea is a potent reliever of heartburn and a great general digestive aid. Meadowsweet tea can help neutralise stomach acids and calm spasms. Traditionally marshmallow has been employed in the treatment of both reflux and digestive disorders as it helps provide a protective layer to the stomach and the oesophagus walls. The leaves, roots and flowers can be delivered via teas, decoctions and syrup.

Aloe vera juice can reduce inflammation and soothe irritation, which is beneficial for an oesophagus lining affected by acid erosion, and it also contains enzymes that neutralise stomach acid – just note that it can have a laxative effect. In traditional Chinese medicine astragalus root has many healing applications – notably to stimulate the immune system and support adrenal-gland functions. It is packed with potent polysaccharides, saponins and flavonoids that contribute to digestive health by reducing stomach acidity and increasing the body's metabolic rate, which not only speeds digestion but also promotes the faster and fuller elimination of waste.

Kitchen support

It's the food you eat that sets acid reflux off, so you need to look at making some dietary changes and opting for more alkaline choices (see page 169). Eat more steamed or roasted vegetables, which rarely aggravate acidity – except tomatoes, which are strongly acidic. The less processed your choices the better, as additives often don't help. An apple a day is suitable here, and bananas are natural antacids too. Pineapple contains bromelain, an enzyme that helps regulate levels of hydrochloric acid in your gastric juices, so do eat more fresh fruits – just be careful with fruit juice, which can be acidic in nature. Vegetable juice, however, is mostly alkaline. Often the advice is to avoid spicy foods but cinnamon, ginger, turmeric and garlic all aid the functioning of the digestion process, slow acidic build-up and limit regurgitation.

Baking soda (sodium bicarbonate) is a base and so cancels out acidity – half a teaspoon well stirred into a small glass of water is the method of delivery. It is not suitable for chronic or prolonged reflux, more a reliever of short-term reflux or heavy meal-triggered heartburn. It contains too much salt for using beyond a week, but you can take the solution five times in a twenty-four-hour period for five days. With prolonged episodes of reflux you might want to consider fighting fire with a type of fire – or should I say acidity with some kitchen acidity. Apple cider vinegar is actually an acidic compound and on paper it would seem like the wrong choice to introduce to a stomach leaking its acidic juices, but it has a powerful role in regulating pH. Amazingly the vinegar actually nudges the stomach towards an alkaline environment by signalling that there is enough acidity present.

A Tropical Beach Soothie Smoothie

Coconut water is alkaline and rich in potassium to soothe an upset stomach. Bananas and melons are antacids. Pineapple regulates levels of hydrochloric acid in your gastric juices. Oats are restorative and energising.

Ingredients

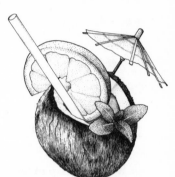

- ½ cup coconut water
- 1 banana
- ½ cup diced pineapple
- ½ cup melon or cantaloupe
- 2 tablespoons oats

Method

Blitz together all the ingredients. Chill before serving and use the same day.

Visualisation to Diminish Stress

Give your stressed system a two-minute vacation. As you sip your delicious tropical smoothie, picture yourself on a tropical beach: the sun setting into the warm ocean, the waves gently lapping against your feet, all the worries of the world lifted from your shoulders. Feel good; feel the warmth on your face, a cool breeze on your neck, the water at your toes, the tropical taste on your tongue. In this way you are programming your brain to help your body feel good.

ANAEMIA

For some anaemia is a persistent or recurring lifelong condition; for others it may be experienced as a once-off dietary deficiency. Anaemia is commonly thought of as an iron deficiency – in fact it is a decrease in your red blood-cell count, or compromised haemoglobin content in the blood (which is dependent on sufficient iron but also B vitamins). Anaemia presents with pallor, fatigue, dizziness and a feeling of being under the weather or generally lacking in vitality. The red cells carry oxygen to the brain and vital organs, so if you are anaemic you are not at your required operating level.

Women need more iron than men. On average an adult woman (19–50) will require 14.8mg per day, while an adult man (19+) will require 8.7mg per day. Many women experience anaemic symptoms around menstruation.

Garden treatments

Sometimes a weed can come to the rescue, and a salad of dandelion greens or chickweed can help you maintain good levels of iron. Alternately you could avail of 1 teaspoon of tincture of yellow dock root (three times daily). Other herbal staples for anaemia include alfalfa, burdock root and the iron-rich nettle – but

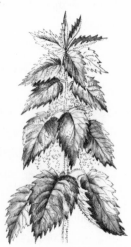

Nettle

any increase in edible plants will help. Chlorophyll is the lifeblood of plants and is compositionally close to the haemoglobin of red blood cells, so consumption of edible foliage makes for a temporary replacement until your body is able to replenish it naturally. Fresh thyme is excellent as a tea or in a soup or casserole, but dried thyme is perhaps one of the most iron-rich herbs you can pluck from the spice rack. One teaspoon of dried thyme delivers around 1.2mg of iron.

Kitchen support

In holistic circles there is often a belief in a kind of sympathetic magic, and many practitioners may suggest that eating red will increase red blood cells, but green might just be the better option. That said, I cannot praise beetroot enough for raising our own internal red. Beetroot boosts oxygen supply and delivery and can support a healthy blood count with its nutritional and phytochemical composition. Of course you should increase iron-rich foods such as salad greens, leafy vegetables, brown rice, lentils and dried fruits (raisins and prunes); bran flakes or fortified cereal are options too. Be sure to cook in iron and not aluminium pots (metal ions infuse into boiling water at cooking temperatures).

B vitamins are good for the blood but folate in particular is necessary for the formation of red blood cells. Folate-rich foods include dark leafy veg and fruits – particularly papaya, oranges, grapefruit and grapes. Folates are also prevalent in beans, so try the following (in order of folate intensity): mung beans, pinto beans, chickpeas, lima beans, black beans, navy beans and kidney beans. Lentils are also excellent. Then there is the option of some asparagus soup – eating just one cup of boiled asparagus delivers approximately 260 micrograms of folic acid, so blitzing that into a soup amalgamates the nutrients that have leached into the cooking water and delivers even more.

Dandelion and Beetroot Salad

The betacyanin pigment that gives beetroot its colour is a powerful antioxidant and blood tonic. Dandelion leaves are a natural spring salad leaf packed with iron and B vitamins. Later in the year simply blanch them (immerse in boiling water for 20 to 30 seconds) to remove the acrid taste that develops with maturity.

Method

For beetroot prep, simply wash off any soil, no need to peel. Place in a pot and cover with water. Boil until tender (when a knife easily slides through), which usually takes an hour to an hour and a half depending on size. Drain. The skins will slide off easily while still warm. Cool, cube and add to your dandelion leaves with any of your favourite salad ingredients – feta cheese, red onion, garlic-brushed bruschetta cubes: whatever you fancy. Remember beetroot tops make good salad greens too.

Feel-good Vinaigrette

An iron-rich salad dressing.

Ingredients

- 2 tablespoons fresh or dried thyme
- 2 tablespoons red wine vinegar
- 2 tablespoons balsamic vinegar
- 8 tablespoons olive oil
- 1 teaspoon honey

Method

Simply combine the thyme and vinegars in a jar or bottle, swirl a little, cover and allow to sit for 10–15 minutes. Then add the oil and honey and shake well before serving. This will last for up to six months in the cupboard.

BACKACHE

There are several types, locations and levels of severity of back-ache. Most are triggered by a pull, a bad night's sleeping position, a lifting error, or a miscalculated movement, and easily resolved with a change of activity and the application of heat. However, some aches can signify a more pronounced injury (slipped discs, torn ligaments, etc.) that will require recuperation and the atten-tion of a medical professional.

The two most commonly experienced backaches are lumbar and thoracic – often the location indicates the injury type: strain and pinched nerve respectively. Depending upon the depth of pain, a rub to flush some blood into the muscle involved and a 'walk-off' may just do the trick. But if it is inflamed and walking is not an option, then an ice pack will be required to reduce swelling and numb the pain. There are also kitchen and garden options to deaden pain.

Lumbar or lower back pain is the most common type of back-ache, especially for gardeners, as that region is the hinge of the majority of our gardening activities. The lumbar region itself is hinged by five vertebrae that act to support the entire weight of your upper body. That weight is added to any incorrect postural stance when strimming, pruning roses or digging over, and it compounds strain when you bend awkwardly or lift incorrectly. Ergonomic posture is vital to avoid backache becoming a regular feature of your gardening activities.

Thoracic or upper and middle back pain is rarer, or at least rarely to do with action injuries (bending awkwardly or lifting incorrectly). The vertebrae here, known as the thoracic vertebrae, are not required to move and flex as the lumbar vertebrae are, and the ache, which can range from dulled stiffness to a sharp or burning sensation, is more likely the result of a pinched nerve or referred lung or rib pain. That said, poor task-posture can trigger upper and middle back pain, so when trimming the top of a hedge or doing a similar chore, do try to keep your back as straight as possible, always balance your weight evenly on both feet and take frequent breaks.

Garden treatments

Many garden plants can be utilised as natural pain relief in tea and tincture form, including angelica, bay, birch, lavender, motherwort, meadowsweet, peppermint, skullcap, St John's wort and, of course, willow bark. Some herbalists recommend internal and external application of horse chestnut extract (see page 252), which is beneficial for lower and sacroiliac/sciatica pain. While a topical gel is easily made from the garden, if you're a novice to herbalism I recommend you purchase horse chestnut tincture from a health store. Valerian is a muscle relaxant that also interrupts and reduces the transmission of pain signals – take this as a tea.

Supplement forms of black cohosh, black haw and devil's claw are popular for their anti-inflammatory and antispasmodic effects. In Chinese traditional medicine both corydalis and dong quai relieve muscular spasms and inflammation. Many over-the-counter creams and rubs for back pain contain methyl salicylates from the mint family, or directly employ arnica, eucalyptus, rosemary or wintergreen.

Kitchen support

Start with some ice, as it will cool the inflammation and slow pain signals. When applying an ice pack always wrap it in a towel or cloth to avoid direct skin contact. Never use ice packs for more than 20 minutes at a time. Breaks of 30–45 minutes between icing periods are advised. Cold therapy only works on day one, so if the pain or ache is still there the next day, swap to heat packs or counterirritant salves for warm relief therapy.

Simply rubbing the affected area introduces a flush of oxygenated blood and helps decrease inflammation and pain signals, but a rub with the lubrication of some coconut oil brings the pain-relieving agent of lauric acid into play. You can add a pinch of cayenne pepper for some heat and the absorption of its pain-relieving capsaicin content. Drinking a teaspoon of cayenne in water, coconut milk or pineapple juice can turn down pain receptors. Coconut meal is also somewhat anti-inflammatory, as is the bromelain content of pineapple flesh – maybe a tropical fruit salad would hit the spot.

Capsicum and Ginger Hot Rub

Chilli spice stimulates endorphin release, even when absorbed through skin, and, like ginger, is topically analgesic and anti-inflammatory. Use as a massaging agent over the affected area. This warm rub flushes blood to sore spots and is easily washed off after treatment.

Method
Mix a teaspoon each of dried chilli flakes and ground ginger with 2 tablespoons of coconut oil.

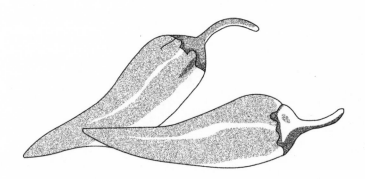

Chillies

Wintergreen Extract Cooling Rub

The foliage of wintergreen is packed full of the pain-relieving, cooling and anti-inflammatory methyl salicylate and using alcohol as a menstruum (to extract the phytochemicals) makes it a rubbing alcohol or liniment base. Witch hazel or vinegar can also be used for extraction.

Method

To make a wintergreen extract simply gather enough foliage to fill a small jam jar or container. Tear each leaf as you place it in. Cover with vodka, put on the lid, shake and allow to infuse for a month inside a dark cupboard. Thereafter, strain off the solids and utilise as a medicated rubbing alcohol. This will keep for up to two years.

CANDIDA

INTESTINAL

Candida is a form of yeast naturally present in our mouth and intestines to expedite both digestion and nutrient absorption. It can, however, be overproduced from time to time.

Garden treatments

Berberine – found in extracts of barberry, goldenseal and Oregon grape root – has a long history of use in traditional Chinese medicine to stimulate the immune system to fight and protect against yeast and fungal infections. It exhibits substantial antifungal activity but it leaves the beneficial microflora in the gut intact. It also prevents candida yeasts from producing lipase – the enzyme that enables their gastrointestinal colonisation.

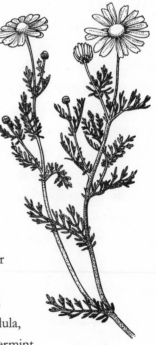

Chamomile

Other garden-grown antifungal herbs include thyme, oregano, calendula, chamomile, fennel, basil, sage, peppermint and rosemary. All make pleasant herbal teas but can also be used in culinary applications – in flavoured vinegars, in infused oils for salad dressings and in soups, stews, casseroles and even sandwiches. A boost in raw foods and salads can help invigorate your good intestinal flora.

Kitchen support

A good place to start is by eliminating sugar and, for a few days to two weeks, lowering your carbohydrate intake to help your system naturally reboot. Eating raw garlic is highly toxic to candida and deeply beneficial to overall human health. This may seem daunting, but it is easy to add to dips, couscous or even rubbed on toast and it brings with it not just antifungal sulphur compounds but also phytoconstituents that promote beneficial gastrointestinal microbes. Garlic supplements or capsules are also good and may even get to your gut more intact.

Natural yoghurt will help bolster those beneficial gastro-intestinal microbes and lessen the spread of infection while, at the other end of the spectrum, apple cider vinegar can attack candida directly. Similarly coconut oil – rich in caprylic acid – directly attacks the cellular structure of yeast. The oleuropein in olive oil and olive leaf extract boosts our systems' ability to fight fungal infections and actively tackles candida overgrowth.

Coconut Oil, Apple Cider and Garlic Vinaigrette

A simple way to deplete candida and harmonise gut flora.

Ingredients
- 1 teaspoon melted/soft coconut oil
- ⅓ cup olive oil
- ⅓ cup apple cider vinegar
- 2 cloves of garlic (deskinned and diced finely)
- A twist of black pepper

Method
Muddle all of the ingredients in a bowl, cover and let sit for an hour to infuse. Decant to a bottle, shake well and cover. This is great over salads and raw food lunches. This type of dressing will naturally separate, so shake well before use.

VAGINAL

Candida is naturally present on human skin and inside the vagina. The normal pH for the vagina is between 3.5 and 4.5, which is acidic, creating an environment where most bacteria can't survive long. So for the most part candida is naturally checked by the vagina's own regulating pH. But when that acid level drops – triggered by menstruation, antibiotic use or other factors – then the yeast population can rise to infection levels. Burning sensations or itches are symptomatic. Discharge and swelling can be present.

Garden treatments

While douching (rinsing or flushing with water or other solutions) is not recommended as a regular practice for a healthy vagina, in this circumstance douches and sipped teas of rosemary, thyme, echinacea and Oregon grape root are traditional treatments to diminish yeast expansion and boost the immune system. Because a douche may spread rather than flush the infection, the stronger the antibacterial herb the better. Goldenseal, with an ethnobotanical history of being used internally as an antifungal agent, can be used as a topical skin rinse or douche application – it has an amazing ability to disrupt fungus from adhering to or entering new host cells. Other potent antifungal herbs include tea tree, burdock, bee balm, calendula, lavender, thyme and uva ursi. Do not substitute any of these herbs with essential oil versions.

Cat's claw, available in your local health store, has been utilised in Peruvian ethno-pharmacology for thousands of years to boost the immune system. One of its active principles is oxindole alkaloids, which enhance phagocytosis (from the Ancient Greek meaning 'to devour'), boosting the way antibodies engulf and destroy pathogens. Other immune-boosting herbs, including astragalus, gingko, hyssop, sage and St John's wort, can get your own healing capacity into gear.

Kitchen support

The aim is to get back to the right pH, so drinking acidic cranberry juice helps. Avoid sugary foods and eat more pro-biotic foods. Eating natural yoghurt and garlic can diminish any candida expansion in the stomach and so give the body a chance to fight off the infection. I would not recommend garlic paste or clove inserts for this ailment – although in theory they would kill off bacteria and yeast, in reality there might be more sting than zing. Bathing externally with a dilution of apple cider vinegar, or adding a cup to your bath, introduces antibacterial and antifungal action, can help address pH and is less likely to sting.

Apple Cider Vinegar Douche

Traditionally utilised to treat bacteria and restore pH.

Method
Simply dilute 2 tablespoons of apple cider vinegar in half a cup of warm water. Use morning and evening until pH is restored.

Apple cider vinegar is a great extraction liquid for the other healing herbs mentioned in the 'Garden treatments' section.

Cranberry, Calendula and Orange Juiced Immune Boost

Between them, cranberries and oranges have plenty of vitamin C to boost the immune system, but on the way out both are tonic and disinfecting to the urinary system. Calendula petals are bacteriostatic (stop bacteria from multiplying) and richly antioxidant (improving blood flow and immune response).

Ingredients
- 1 cup fresh cranberries
- 2 oranges
- 4–5 calendula flower heads

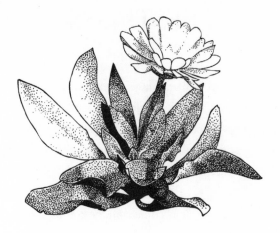

Calendula

Method

We don't just want the juice here – we want the fibre too. So wash
the cranberries, peel the oranges, wash the flower heads and pick
off the petals to use. Add all to the blender as you go. Hit the
button. Chill and enjoy.

CHESTINESS

Chestiness can result from mucus formation causing congestion, or a bacterial infection bringing about wheezing and impaired breathing function. It can accompany a common cold or be a symptom of an underlying medical condition. A GP visit is worthwhile to clarify.

Congested chest: this may come with the common cold or in the form of a 'winter chest', when the elements and the temperature fluctuation of home/office and garden/outside seem to offset our immune responses. See also sinusitis (page 219). Summer congestion can be due to seasonal allergies (see page 145) or a summer cold.

Chest infection/upper respiratory tract infection: what we typically think of as a chest infection is often an upper respiratory tract infection (URTI). URTIs can affect the nasal passage and sinuses, the pharynx and larynx too. Chest infections can come via a cold or flu, or as a standalone infection. There are two main approaches – killing the infection (with antibacterial herbs and herbs to boost our immune system) and clearing or expelling the infection (with decongestants and mucus-busting herbs).

Garden treatments

Inhaling the scent of a few peppermint leaves, rolled or crushed between your hands to release all the decongestant menthol-like vapours, helps soothe and clear both congestion and the mind.

Those same vapours can make a wonder salve to see you right if a winter chest or summer-cold-triggered congestion is slowing your enjoyment of the garden or impeding daily life. Peppermint tea is also excellent to relieve and support. Eucalyptus leaves contain the aromatic volatile oil eucalyptol, which is decongestant in both aromatherapeutic and salve format.

Marshmallow root and leaf tea or tincture can loosen phlegm and ease coughs, while mullein is expectorant and soothing. Elderberry and echinacea are both antiviral and anti-inflammatory. Goldenseal is known to calm inflamed mucous membranes and also stimulates the production of white blood cells to fight off any viral or bacterial infection. Mullein is antibacterial and antiviral and is an expectorant. Lungwort was once popular for respiratory care, as its lung-shaped leaves made it a candidate for treatment of that part of the body in medical herbalism – if it looked like the part, it might cure the part. It was also utilised to clear congestion of the chest. Scientifically it does contain antibiotic phytochemicals and antibacterial principles useful in disarming respiratory infections. Coltsfoot (tincture or tea) has been long used to clear excess mucus from the lungs and bronchial tubes. Likewise thyme – in tea or tincture form – can assist clearance and also fight the infection. Echinacea works by boosting our own production of properdin/factor P – a sort of immune-catalyst – and so supports our antibodies to fight infection rapidly.

Kitchen support

A quick kitchen cure is to chop some fresh ginger into boiling water and infuse for 10–20 minutes to yield a strong ginger tea;

add a teaspoon of honey to each cup as you sip throughout the day. Together the honey and ginger assist in loosening the mucus and soothing the throat and chest. Garlic also opens airways and flushes toxins from the blood. Sage tea, which is a traditional treatment for sore throats and stubborn coughs, can be used in steam inhalations to clear chest infections, thanks to its camphor and salvene content. Garlic, ginger and sage can also be added to your dinner. Mint, and its menthol content, is great in inhalations, and when added to food or juices it opens up the respiratory system and enables free breathing. You could try a mucus-cleansing diet and decrease mucus production with citrus fruits, apricots, peaches, plums, root and leaf vegetables, onions, garlic, horseradish, chickpeas, celery, parsley, watercress and pine nuts.

Clove and Mint Chest Rub

Mint yields menthol, which is analgesic, cooling and counter-irritant, as well as vasodilating. The aroma and phytochemical actions of the clove also boost the 'breathe easier' sensation of this treatment.

Ingredients
- ½ cup sunflower oil
- 1 teaspoon ground cloves or 20 drops clove essential oil
- 1 cup peppermint foliage (or other culinary mint)
- 25g unadulterated beeswax
- Water

Method

Bring a saucepan of water to the boil. Add the sunflower oil and cloves to a mason jar, put on the lid and sit it into the saucepan of hot water. Wash and kitchen-towel dry the mint leaves, then tear or roughly chop to release their active principles as you add them to the warm oil. Replace the lid on the jar. Bring the water to the boil again – to heat the oil and help extract the phytochemicals – then simmer for 20 minutes. Allow the jar to rest off the heat for a further 20 minutes. Strain the herb parts away, then bring the water around the oil-filled jar to the boil again and chip, shave or grate the beeswax into the infused oil and stir until it dissolves fully and ameliorates. Finally, decant the mixed liquid into your storage container and allow to cool and solidify before sealing and storing for use. This rub is intended for massage application to the chest and back. It is suitable for inhalation and vaporising, or steam-bath inhalation – it is not for consumption. Keeps for up to a year.

COLD AND FLU

OK, how do you know if it's a cold or the flu? Most over-the-counter treatments claim to tackle both colds and flu, and so we often think of the flu as a stronger version of a cold, or the common cold as a type of flu. The truth is they do have similar symptoms – congestion (see page 60), sore throat (see page 223) and sneezing, but they are different viral infections. The flu, apart from exhibiting these shared symptoms with more intensity, is also attended by a high fever, body aches, weakness and fatigue (see page 123). Colds develop slowly but flu symptoms are much more abrupt and debilitating.

THE COMMON COLD/RHINOVIRUSES

A cold is really an immune-system reaction to an airborne viral infection of the nose and throat – hence its medical definition as a rhinovirus (rhino for nose and not for the sensation, sometimes accompanying, that you have been hit by a charging rhino). Sneezing, runny nose, coughing and a sore throat are symptomatic. It can also occasion congestion of the chest and fatigue. While there is no cure, there are plenty of options for alleviation of symptoms. Rest, hydration and immune support is the best course of treatment to tackle the causative factor of a rhinovirus. Colds typically last from three to ten days, with an incubation period of two to three days before that first sniffle or scratchy throat.

Garden treatments

Peppermint tea is stimulating and pain relieving and works to alleviate many of the ancillary symptoms too. Meadowsweet tea can address pains and fevers. Elderberry is particularly effective against respiratory viral infections and will boost overall immunity as it is also loaded with vitamin C. Thyme stimulates the production of infection-destroying white blood cells. In terms of a little garden aromatherapy, inhaling thyme, sage, peppermint, rosemary, lavender and eucalyptus can help clear congestion and also address tiredness and poor concentration.

Kitchen support

Consume more citrus fruits for their vitamin C and its infection-busting potential. Zinc, in nuts and pumpkin seeds, acts similarly. Ginger, honey, garlic and black pepper can all help fight off infections and soothe symptoms. Barley water (see page 69) is a healthy beverage. But best of all is green tea, which, apart from being antioxidant and rejuvenating, actually stimulates the liver to secrete interferon – a most potent anti-infection agent.

Immuno-Catalyst Honey and Lemon Syrup

Does what it says on the tin.

Method

Simply mix equal parts of lemon juice and honey by volume and fold into yoghurt or use as the base of a cordial or hot beverage (simply add sparkling or hot water).

Roasted Tomato and Thyme Soup

Beyond vitamin C, tomato soup also supplies vitamins A, E and K and the disease-fighting goodness of lycopene. Thyme is a natural flavour companion to tomato and also an immunity booster.

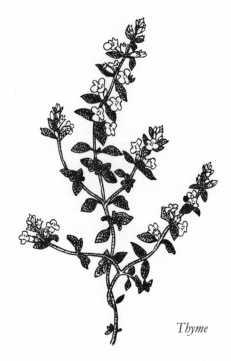

Thyme

Ingredients

- 1lb ripe tomatoes (any variety but the redder they are the more lycopene they contain)
- 1 tablespoon olive oil
- 2 tablespoons chopped fresh thyme

- ½ cup water or vegetable stock
- 1 clove garlic
- Salt and pepper to season

Method

Preheat the oven to 190°C (375°F/Gas Mark 5). Roughly chop the tomatoes and place in a roasting tin. Drizzle the olive oil over the tomatoes and swirl to coat. Place in the oven for 30 minutes. Meanwhile boil the thyme in the water or vegetable stock, then remove from the heat. Pour the thyme-infused liquid and cooked tomatoes into a blender. Add the garlic, peeled and finely chopped. Blitz to a smooth texture. Add salt and pepper to taste, serve and enjoy. This reheats well and, if making larger servings, it will keep in the fridge for up to three days.

INFLUENZA

Flu is caused by the airborne influenza A, B or C virus infecting the upper and lower respiratory tract. With virus C we self-immunise against repeat infections, but A and B are constantly mutating and so can be contracted repeatedly. Incubation is typically one to two days. Symptoms last two to five days. They include fever (see page 133), headache (see page 149), aches and pains (see page 36), chills, sore throat (see page 223), cough (see page 79), nausea and vomiting (see page 204), dehydration and sometimes diarrhoea (see page 95).

When we get the flu, our immune system dispatches two types of white blood cells. The first type are called T and B lymphocytes, which support antibodies to wrap themselves around the virus and prevent it from adhering to a cell wall or replicating itself. The second type – known as a macrophage – will ingest and destroy the debilitated virus. Many of the herbs below boost that activity.

Garden treatments

Smell lavender for its irritability-reducing values and its decongestant principles, or inhale eucalyptus for a clearing effect. Sage tea is helpful for many of the symptoms, such as sweating, chills and sore throat, but really we want to boost our immunity with echinacea, astragalus, elderflower, elderberry, chamomile and juniper berries. Other botanical antivirals include goldenseal, milk thistle, pau d'arco and St John's wort. Gargling with cooled thyme tea helps kill off residual viruses and soreness in the mouth and throat. Thyme contains the antimicrobial thymol and the antiviral thujanol – both amazing at halting flu viruses in their tracks – and thyme has an affinity with white blood cells, boosting their production and efficiency.

Kitchen support

Sometimes a cup of tea is all you need – sipping tea hydrates, eases stomach discomfort and helps calm over-worked mucous membranes. Tea's antioxidants give the body a boost towards recovery too. With green tea, two catechins, epicatechin-gallate (ECG) and epigallocatechin-gallate (EGCG), actively inhibit the reproduction and replication ability of the influenza virus. Make a pot with some of the herbs mentioned above added.

Barley water is good to reduce a fever and settle the stomach.

Hot lemon and honey is antiviral and energy boosting. To boost immune-system responses eat plenty of vitamin-C-rich foods and plenty of zinc-rich foods. Consider the medicinal mushrooms (see page 131) and also the antiviral and system-strengthening staples of garlic, cinnamon, turmeric and ginger. Ginger tea or grated ginger in meals can help the body perspire and eliminate toxins, but it also helps with stomach upset and fatigue. One apple has an antioxidant effect within the human body equivalent to 1,500mg of vitamin C. Soaking in a soothing bath of apple cider vinegar and Epsom salt (one-third of a cup of each) eliminates toxins and refreshes tired muscles.

Barley Water

There are two options for making barley water. You can slowly infuse it overnight, or you can bring all the ingredients to a boil, allow to cool, strain away the solids and have a same-day barley water. Both are tasty and healing beverages and can be stored for three days if refrigerated.

Ingredients
- 1 cup organic pearl barley
- 1 litre water
- ½ lemon

Method
To a large jug add the pearl barley, the water and the lemon zest

and juice. Stir well. Cover with a tea towel and allow to soak until the same time next day in the fridge or on a countertop. Strain away the solids and chill to serve. Sweeten to taste if desired.

Echinacea and Thyme Flu Buster (a quick blitz tincture)

For internal immunity boosting and external antimicrobial action.

Ingredients
- ½ cup echinacea (root is best but leaves, stems and flowers are all valuable for extracting immune-stimulant and anti-microbial agents)
- ½ cup thyme leaves
- 500ml vodka or brandy

Method
Blitz all the ingredients in a blender – as fine as possible – pour into a jar, cover and place in a sunny window, to be shaken daily for a week. You can dip in then, but preferably let it sit for a second week and then strain away the solids and bottle up.

Dosage and duration
10–25 drops of the tincture, three times daily for five days, with a short break of two days before the second round.

COLD SORES
(*HERPES SIMPLEX LABIALIS*)

A cold sore manifests as a small blister or cluster of blisters occurring on the lips (and sometimes also the face). It is caused by a viral infection – herpes simplex virus type 1 (HSV-1). Tingling, itching or burning sensations generally herald the blistering to come. As a virus it is highly contagious and has its own life cycle. Some people get a cold sore once and it never returns but, with most, once contracted the virus remains for many years, if not for a lifetime. Thankfully it is predominantly dormant with possibly one or two flare-ups each year, but it is also easily triggered into activity by sunburn or other damage to the lip surface and also by stress or fatigue. So looking after yourself is the best way to keep it repressed.

Outbreaks generally clear up without any intervention or treatment within seven to ten days. There are plenty of over-the-counter lip balms and topical creams to suppress the viral activity and soothe the soreness and there are many home cures, too, to make it more manageable.

Garden treatments

Topical tincture or tisane rinses of selfheal, goldenseal, St John's wort or hyssop are antiviral. Lavender or thyme in a balm or blitzed into a paste are also beneficial. The juice of houseleeks is soothing and hydrating, which is key to relief. To address the

flare-up try antiviral iced teas harvested from your own garden
– they not only boost your
internal immune system but
also work on contact with the
lips and mouth. I would opt for
chamomile, as it contains bisabolol,
an antimicrobial wound healer, and its
anti-inflammatory nature is beneficial

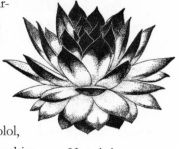

Houseleek

too. You can also try lemon balm, bergamot, mint, echinacea or
thyme. Liquorice root contains glycyrrhizic acid that can inhibit
and fight viral spread.

Kitchen support

Over-the-counter antiviral creams work at the tingle stage but
are generally ineffective thereafter, while honey works at every
stage to suppress the surfacing virus, soothe any pain or itch,
seal bleeding, soften scabs and promote replacement skin cells
at wound sites. A dusting of cinnamon is a great antiseptic and
dries up ruptured blisters and bleeds. One of the best things you
can do is avoid acidic or salty foods, as they not only sting but
also can suppress your immune system just as it attempts to fight
the virus flare-up. The mistake is to reduce eating and drinking
for fear of bursting a blister or cracking a scab – you need to
drink plenty of fluids to keep the lip hydrated and functioning
normally in unaffected areas.

Four Essences Medicated Lip Balm

Vegetable butter and oil are moisturising and absorb the essential oils and their antiviral and healing principles, while the thickening agent – beeswax – is naturally antimicrobial and wound healing.

Ingredients
- 1 tablespoon shea butter or cocoa butter
- 1 tablespoon grated beeswax
- 1 tablespoon olive oil
- 2 shakes each essential oil of lavender, tea tree, thyme and German chamomile

Method
In a bain-marie (or jam jar resting in hot water), melt the shea or cocoa butter and beeswax into the olive oil. Once melted remove from the heat. Stir with a chopstick or swirl around to ameliorate. Add the essential oils at the last minute, just before decanting to a suitable container such as a small glass jar or tin. Cover to retain volatile oils and allow to cool and set naturally. Use as often as you need to soothe and treat. The balm can be stored in a cool place for several months.

Tea Tree

Cold Sore Blitz Paste

All ingredients are antiviral, anti-inflammatory and pain relieving.

Ingredients
- 2 tablespoons coconut oil
- 1 tablespoon lavender foliage
- 1 tablespoon chopped chamomile tops (flowers or foliage)
- 1 teaspoon honey

Method

Simply blitz together all the ingredients. Use as a dab treatment throughout the day, each day until the virus subsides. Stores in the fridge for a week.

CONSTIPATION

A successful bowel movement depends on three factors: peristalsis (the wavelike contraction of smooth muscle in your intestines), fibre and moisture. Constipation is a reduction in the frequency of your normal pattern of bowel movements, the usual frequency varying from person to person and often week to week. Constipation can be 'wanting' to go but it just not happening – or it can be that activity has ground to a halt for a few days or is translating into intermittent and painful defecations rather than regular activity over an extended period. Diet, poor fitness levels, disturbed routine, ill health and some medications can all occasion constipation. It can be a factor of pregnancy. The good news is that it is short term and treatable.

Garden treatments

The potent laxative senna won't grow in every garden but is stocked in health stores – it can be more purgative than gentle, as is the case with aloe and buckthorn. Other milder laxatives include cramp bark, marshmallow root, dandelion root, burdock root and angelica root – all simply taken via a tea. Heartsease is mildly laxative and diuretic. Both milk thistle seed and fennel seed tea are helpful to the digestive system and bowel movements. A salad of chickweed and dandelion foliage with some rosemary vinegar has roots in folk medicine – the ingredients can all stimulate the system and so promote movement. Fenugreek, flaxseed and psyllium seeds are garden and health store staples that act as a herbal bulk laxative – 'bulk' being the physical potential to move things through, not the amount you need to ingest. Mucilage herbs, which have a soothing, gelatinous nature, include marshmallow root and slippery elm bark. An abdominal massage of basil lotion or essential oil blend – in a clockwise direction – is beneficial.

Burdock

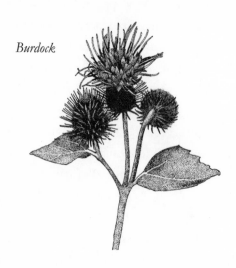

Kitchen support

Insufficient dietary fibre is perhaps the leading cause of or contribution to constipation – so in general more fruit and vegetables and a day started with wholemeal cereals will hasten an end to it. Magnesium can help restore regularity and can be sourced through fruits and veg, and also through apple cider vinegar. Figs, prunes and raisins are all kitchen-cupboard cures for this condition, as they provide bulk, fibre and key vitamins that relax the bowel. Don't forget the benefits of live yoghurt and probiotics to restore intestinal vitality.

Blackberry, Fig, Prune and Raisin Compote

These top fruits with laxative potential make a tasty compote suitable to stir into natural yoghurt (probiotic) or put over muesli (high fibre). For muesli recipes, see pages 127–8.

Ingredients
- 3 prunes
- 3 dried figs
- 1 tablespoon lemon juice
- 1 tablespoon honey
- 6 blackberries
- 1 tablespoon raisins
- 1 tablespoon blackberry jam (or jam of choice)

Method
Pit the prunes. Roughly chop the figs and prunes to raisin size. In a saucepan, heat the lemon juice and honey and bring to a boil, constantly stirring – then add all the fruit and the jam. Stir well. Turn off the heat and allow to fully cool and set. Chill in the fridge, where it will keep for three days. Use as required.

Ocean Motion Isotonic Drink

One of the old folk treatments for constipation was to imbibe some sea water (a natural laxative) to loosen affairs. You don't have to buy a new bucket and spade, or have a repertoire of sea shanties – a glass of tap water with a tablespoon of sea salt from the spice rack will do the trick. This is not for sustained constipation, as salt intake brings other complications with prolonged use. Sometimes the issue is just inadequate fluids, and several cups of water or herbal tea will go a long way to remedy it.

COUGH

A cough is more the consequence of a condition than a condition itself, though we often rush to treat it in isolation from underlying symptoms and triggers. Really a cough is just a natural reaction to irritation of the throat, trachea or bronchial tubes, helping to expel any irritating material or mucus accumulations. Coughing can also be triggered by swallowing dust or animal hairs (whether you're allergic or not), the catching of too dry food or the bronchial impact of cold or infection. Sometimes a glass of water is the cure; other times you need to address the asthma, cold or flu (see page 64) causing the cough. See also chest congestion (page 60).

To deal with the cough itself we have many routes to take, be it prescription, over the counter, herbal or kitchen concocted. To choose the most effective remedies, it's worth understanding the terminology around them. Antitussive means cough suppressant; expectorant means to loosens mucus and expel; demulcents are soothing to irritated bronchial tubes. Many cough sweets and syrups, apart from having a medicinal value (suppressive or expelling), do good by being demulcent.

Garden treatments

The original sign for a pharmacy, before the green cross, was an illustration or carving of coltsfoot. Coltsfoot has a long herbal tradition of suppressing coughs, expelling mucus and soothing irritated membranes, encompassing all the methods of tackling a cough. Heartsease tea is somewhat expectorant and a petal smoothie (a few heads blended with a strawberry and green tea) has both mucilage properties and phytochemicals soothing to the chest. Most herbs are either antitussive or expectorant by action, but also somewhat demulcent in their delivery if used in syrup, saliva-stimulating sweets, etc.; some herbs are particularly demulcent in action too. Those listed here also have, to varying degrees, antibacterial and antiviral properties. Antitussives include coltsfoot, angelica, liquorice, horehound, hyssop, thyme, goldenseal, wild cherry bark, garlic and ginger. Expectorants include elderflower, elecampane root, fennel, fenugreek, black cohosh root, bloodroot, couch grass, slippery elm, peppermint, horseradish root, coltsfoot and speedwell. Demulcent herbs include aloe vera, burdock, marshmallow, couch grass, liquorice, coltsfoot, goldenseal, elecampane, slippery elm and hyssop. Herbs more applicable to dry coughs include mallow, mullein and liquorice root, while mucus or congested coughs benefit from cowslip or thyme added to the preparation of teas, syrups or cough drops.

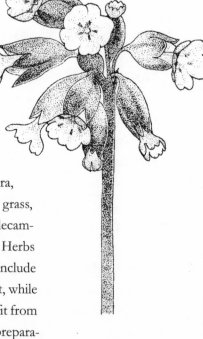

Cowslip

Kitchen support

If you don't fancy the idea of garlic syrup (the immuno-boosting and antibacterial potency of garlic is great to treat the underlying causes of a cough), then a honey and lemon combination is a powerful staple to soothe the throat and boost the immune system. Grapes are somewhat expectorant but also have a tonic effect on your lungs – the juice of grapes can be made into a cough syrup. Raw or cooked onions are recommended for removing phlegm. Aniseed and cinnamon are two good spices to soothe sore throats and alleviate coughing. Any of the herbs listed above can be made into ice pops, granitas, ice-creams or sorbets to cool and soothe, and even mixed with grape, honey or lemon in the process. Homemade lemonade really gets the vitamin C in but, just like iced tea, it cools and hydrates too.

Grape Juice and Honey Cough Syrup

Grape juice and honey are brilliant soothers with clearing potential.

Method

Bring to a frothy boil 3 parts by volume of honey to 1 part by volume of grape juice. Simmer for 5 minutes to reduce. Decant to a container and allow to cool before use. Stores for a week in the fridge. Can be taken from a spoon several times daily to ease symptoms and soothe the throat.

Cough Sucks Cough Drops

The ingredients reduce phlegm, suppress cough spasms and decrease irritation and inflammation.

Ingredients

- ¼ cup grape juice
- ½ teaspoon ground cloves
- ½ teaspoon ground aniseed
- 1 tablespoon lemon juice
- 1 tablespoon honey
- ½ cup granulated sugar
- 2 tablespoons caster sugar
- Parchment paper
- Cornflour

Method

In a saucepan bring the grape juice and spices to a frothy boil, then add the lemon juice, honey and sugar, stirring constantly. Simmer for 10–15 minutes or until a thick syrupy texture forms. Remove from the heat. Spread out a sheet of parchment paper and dust with about a tablespoon of caster sugar. Next simply spoon some drops of the thick syrup onto the sheet to form little buttons. You can dust the tops with the remaining castor sugar or with cinnamon if you prefer. If you are happy with the shapes, simply allow them to fully set into suckable medicated lozenges. Or you can allow them to cool enough to handle and then roll them into balls, or use shaped moulds. The sweets may stick together in warm environments, so a dusting of cornflour after setting will help prevent that.

DERMATOLOGICAL AILMENTS

COMMON ISSUES: DERMATITIS, PSORIASIS AND ECZEMA

Dermatitis is a noncontagious inflammation issue. It has many forms and triggers but the common denominators are an itchy rash or swollen, reddened skin that may blister or ooze, developing a crust and flaking, on the scalp, elbows, hands or body. An irritant or an allergen can trigger dermatitis, but help is available to decrease the fires of inflammation.

Eczema is thought to be a reaction to environmental irritants or allergies and is not contagious. Commonly first experienced in infancy, it often resolves between five years of age and just before adolescence. For some it can follow into adulthood. Certainly, for those who have not shaken the condition by adolescence, its symptoms are worsened by both stress and hormonal fluctuations. Outbreaks include dry, itchy, inflamed and red-blotched skin, which will often flake or crack. Avoid scratching and excessive rubbing to limit secondary complications such as these.

Psoriasis is a chronic inflammatory, non-contagious skin disease. The condition accelerates the rate at which skin cells are produced, turned over and shed from the skin from a normal monthly cycle to a weekly one or even shorter. That fast turnover results in blotching, scaling and discomfort. The name is from the Greek word *psōra* meaning itch – the name is apt. Most people develop psoriasis in their teens or early twenties or, later in life, after fifty. There are a few forms, but the most common is known as plaque psoriasis, which manifests as distinctive patches of raised reddish skin, covered with a whitish silver layer that eventually scales. Outbreaks are prominent at elbows, knees, scalp and lower back.

Garden treatments

UV rays are still considered a very effective treatment for eczema and psoriasis, so a little garden sun is good and much better than a tanning bed. Avoiding harsh chemical- and soap-based cleansers is essential to let the skin recover – so washes, cleansers and lotions can be made from heartsease, calendula, chamomile, field scabious, slippery elm, burdock, red clover, cleavers and chickweed. Dermatitis can be an allergic reaction to fabric softener or shower gel or, heaven forbid, a plant in the garden (I explore garden-generated dermatitis and allergic contact conditions in detail in *First Aid from the Garden*), but until you discover your plant sensitivities it is best to use vinegar rinses as a non-steroidal anti-inflammatory to soothe the reaction. Psoriasis benefits from vinegar and home remedies (this is covered extensively in *Beauty Treatments from the Garden*), but gamma-linolenic acid (GLA)

Calendula

from evening primrose and other garden sources is very effective in slowing the shedding rate – topically applied and also taken internally in supplement form.

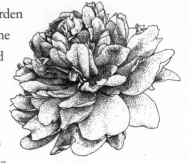

For all of these conditions, aloe vera gel and strawberry pulp both cool and soothe flared skin at the moment of irritation, while oolong tea or

Peony

red peony tea can be taken orally or utilised as a bathing solution to address derma inflammation. Chickweed and calendula are two excellent skin-healing agents. The astringency of witch hazel is also beneficial. Poultices of dock leaf and cabbage pastes are old folk cures.

Kitchen support

Topical applications of coconut oil can, for many, reduce redness and dryness/scaling within a couple of days and the lauric acid content of the oil is pain-relieving, antimicrobial and stimulates an effective immune response. The oleic acid and omega-9 fatty acids in olive oil, if added to your diet, can suppress inflammation and flare-ups. Think also of foods that contain psoralen, a compound that supports the body's own defences against psoriasis and eczema. Psoralen-rich foods include figs, fennel, carrots, celery, celeriac, coriander, parsnips and parsley. Apple cider vinegar is a non-steroidal anti-inflammatory that also helps resolve scales and itchiness, while oatmeal is soothing and moisturising, as is honey.

Borage Skin-Replenishing Cream

This contains GLA and moisturising ingredients to alleviate and treat a broad array of skin complaints.

Ingredients
- 1 tablespoon chopped borage flowers
- 2 tablespoons olive oil
- 1 tablespoon borage or evening primrose oil
- ½ tablespoon grated beeswax
- ½ tablespoon grated/granulated emulsifying wax
- 3–4 tablespoons witch hazel extract

Method

Add the flowers and oils to a bain-marie, bring the water to the boil, then turn off the heat – rest for an hour to infuse. Reheat and add the waxes. Keep the heat on until they are fully melted, then remove from the heat and slowly add the witch hazel – spoon by spoon – whisking as you go. Allow the mixture to cool for 20 minutes, then whisk to a creamy consistency. This will keep for six months.

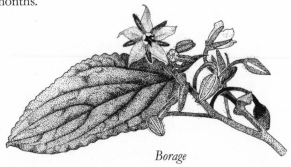

Borage

Oatmeal and Oolong Tea Bath Soak

A skin-soothing and remedial soak with a silky dimension.

Ingredients
- Flaked oats
- Oolong tea

Method
The ratio by volume is 1 part tea to 3 parts oats. Add to a food processor and pulse to a fine powder. Add a few tablespoons to running bathwater. This keeps well for months in airtight, dry containers.

Oatmeal and oolong tea shower wash – to make a shower version simply add ½ cup of powdered oatmeal and oolong to 1 cup of Castile soap and stir well – milkiness is a good sign. Decant to storage containers and use as a shower gel. This keeps for several weeks.

MINOR DERMATOLOGICAL ISSUES: RASHES, HIVES AND ITCHY SKIN

Some of these ailments are symptoms of psoriasis, dermatitis and eczema, but others are standalone ailments in themselves, spontaneous or allergic reactions that can appear from nowhere and linger or go just as quickly – there are, of course, natural ways to speed up their exit.

Rashes are for the most part allergic reactions or infection indicators that manifest at skin level with inflammation and discolouration – so while we may treat these with antihistamines and anti-inflammatories, it is important to trace the source of the irritation. Some rashes are a contact dermatitis or the result of fungal, bacterial, parasitic or viral infection. They can clear up quickly, but any rashes lasting more than a few days (especially if unexplained) should be evaluated by a medical professional.

Take all childhood rashes seriously. If worried, conduct the glass test – roll a glass tumbler over the rash. If it is an infection of meningococcal bacteria (which can lead to meningitis and septicaemia), it will not fade under the pressure of the glass and the next step is to call an ambulance. Less harmful rashes are more minor skin irritations and are easily treated or alleviated with kitchen and garden remedies.

Hives (*urticaria*) are in the category of rash. They manifest as sudden outbreaks of red, generally itchy, spots or welts on the skin. It is often called nettle rash, as it resembles the rash caused by an encounter with nettles – this is evident too in its medical name of 'urticaria', the botanical name for the nettle being *Urtica dioica*. The rash is due to histamine production, which indicates an allergic response. Pollen, plant sap, spores, insects, dander, some chemicals, soaps and a large range of garden-encountered substances and household products can trigger histamine to be released by cells in the skin, causing blood vessels to dilate and leak fluid out onto the skin surface. This oedema is the basis of the hive/rash/urticaria. Hives usually go within twenty-four hours, but longer-lasting bouts are considered chronic urticaria and require antihistamines and a care regime.

Garden treatments

Rosemary tea, cooled, acts as a topical non-steroidal, anti-inflammatory wash – fresh sprigs added to vinegar can be utilised as a spritz. Antihistamines for topical application include basil, baical skullcap, chamomile, coltsfoot, houseleek, goldenseal, mint and thyme. Antihistamines for internal consumption include burdock, elderberry, gingko, nettle, chamomile, echinacea, cat's claw, parsley and thyme.

Kitchen support

Start with a cup of green tea – it contains two antihistamine compounds, quercetin and catechins. Then have a snack of some foods with reaction-reducing vitamin C and strong antihistamine action such as bananas, bell peppers, broccoli, Brussels sprouts, cauliflower, kale, kohlrabi, kiwi fruit, guavas, gooseberries, strawberries, pineapples, papayas and melons. Omega-3 fatty acids and vitamin A are beneficial in reducing allergic reactions.

Quercetin is also found in broccoli, bell peppers, berries, red onions, garlic and red apples. A smear of honey is always good as a skin tonic and its antimicrobial action may hit the spot.

Chamomile, Milk and Honey Lotion

All the ingredients work to reduce skin inflammation and neutralise the histamine or defence reaction caused by nettle rash, nettle sting, heat rash, sunburn and other irritations that trigger body rashes. Zinc is antipruritic (stops itching).

Ingredients
- ½ cup chamomile flowers/tops
- ½ cup coconut or almond milk
- ½ cup pre-made strong chamomile tea
- 2 tablespoons zinc ointment or 1 crushed zinc tablet
- 2 tablespoons baking soda
- 2 tablespoons honey

Method
Soak the chamomile flowers/tops in the milk overnight, then strain out the flowers and combine with all the other ingredients in a bowl. Whisk well (if using a hand blender you can leave the flowers in). Apply as needed to the affected area of skin. Keep refrigerated and use within five days.

Itchy skin (*pruritus*) can manifest as a reaction to an allergen or a consequence of dermatitis, psoriasis or eczema. Scratching can sometimes exacerbate it – so resist if you can. Emollients are often the first line of treatment for pruritus. The herbs mentioned below can be utilised (infused or blended) with emollients to deliver a medicated application.

Garden treatments

Both aloe vera and houseleek sap can cool and resolve itching skin. Heartsease is tonic to skin and was once popularly sipped to quell skin eruptions; it is also excellent as a topical wash. Chamomile tea to drink helps de-stress the immune system, or it can be applied as a wash to calm irritation. Simply harvest some flowering tops and a little foliage and infuse in hot water for 5 minutes. Cool sufficiently before drinking or applying to skin. Juniper berries, mint, thyme and rosemary are anti-inflammatory skin soothers. Topically applied, the juices of dock leaf, plantain, chickweed, peppermint and calendula flowers are all antipruritic. Witch hazel is also very effective.

Garden-grown antihistamines such as chamomile, nettle and fennel are also very helpful, as allergic itchiness is triggered by the presence or release of the histamine protein which can easily pass the blood–brain barrier and is implicated

A Dock Leaf

in the communication of inflammation and itch sensations. Antihistamines actively disable the protein, halt the signalling of the itch sensation and stop the brain from making us scratch.

Kitchen support

Oats are soothing to skin and antipruritic. Soak in warm water for an hour, blitz to a lotion and apply to itchy areas. The pH of baking soda also counteracts itchy and troubled skin – it can be added to the oat lotion or made into a paste. Foods that stabilise cells, and so prevent both the production and release of histamine, are apples, berries, broccoli, onions, garlic, parsley, tea, tomatoes, lettuce, legumes and any food with quercetin (bright pigment). Hemp seeds and flaxseed deliver omega-3 fatty acids, which are anti-inflammatory and lessen allergenic reactions.

K-Itch'n No Itch'n Body Mask

To a bowl add 2 tablespoons each of ground cinnamon, honey and baking soda, 1 cup of finely ground oatmeal and 1 cup of soya milk. Mix into a porridge-like consistency or blend with some green tea to make a lotion – apply topically. This is used for instant relief and cannot be stored.

Plantain Paste

A mortar and pestle paste of plantain leaf, a pinch of salt and a drop of water eases swelling and itching. This is used for instant relief and cannot be stored.

The Salt Solution

Make half a cup of strong chamomile or lemon-balm tea or tincture and, instead of sugaring it, add several large spoonfuls of salt and two large spoonfuls of baking soda. Stir well and place in the freezer for a moment or two – until it's cool enough to wash the skin with. This is used for instant relief and cannot be stored.

DIARRHOEA

Increased frequency of defecation or occasions of watery stools can indicate ingestion of toxins or food allergens or contamination (see food poisoning, page 233). It can be a side effect of conventional medication, or be stress or illness related – including irritable bowel syndrome, Crohn's disease or coeliac disease. Mostly it is the result of viral or bacterial infection (see gastro-enteritis page 230). Diarrhoea will cause dehydration and may occasion cramping, nausea (see page 204), bloating/flatulence (see page 104) and general debility. The first aim is to kill off the bacteria or parasite causing the occurrence. The second is to keep hydrated and replace the lost electrolytes and minerals. The third is to calm the stomach. Between garden and kitchen we can easily sort out all three.

Garden treatments

Traditionally astringents (to dry up), such as tormentil tea, raspberry leaf tea or blackberry leaf tea, have been utilised to stop diarrhoea and maintain hydration in the process. Folk cures include dandelion, meadowsweet and shepherd's purse, which all help with digestion and ease cramps too. Antispasmodic herbs include black cohosh, cramp bark, evening primrose oil, motherwort, nettle and valerian. Chamomile tea is soothing to the digestive system, as are fennel, mint and catmint. Herbalists may prescribe astragalus for its antiviral, antibacterial and antimicrobial activities – it also contains polysaccharides that support the immune system. Any of the garden antibiotics such as goldenseal, echinacea or oregano will help tackle the cause.

Kitchen support

The tannins in a simple cup of de-caffeinated tea can reduce spasm, cramp and inflammation. Drink plenty of fluids, but avoid caffeine and alcohol for a time. Ginger, sliced or in tea form, is helpful with upset stomachs and intestinal distress – it alleviates cramps and any accompanying nausea. Ginger ale is a traditional remedy to make stools less watery, while carrot juice is soothing to the system and helps dry up stools. Some

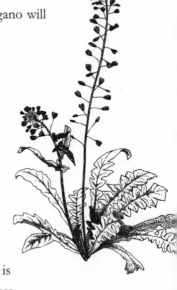

Shepherd's purse

raw garlic for a couple of days can kill off the parasites and bacteria that cause most cases of diarrhoea. Stew some apples or make apple sauce, as the pectin reduces intestinal inflammation – blackberry jam works the same way and if used on brown bread adds some good fibre to the mix. Cinnamon, brewer's yeast and carob powder have a history in treating diarrhoea and can be mixed with apple sauce or jam. Coconut oil contains lauric acid, which, when ingested, delivers antiviral, antimicrobial, antiprotozoal and antifungal properties.

Potassium loss is an issue, so eat more potatoes, squash, beans, dark leafy greens, mushrooms, yoghurt, avocados and bananas.

The digestive-resistant starch of precooked cold potatoes has a health-boosting effect on the intestines – make a potato salad when you're feeling up to eating.

Cinnamon Apple Sauce

Nourishing and soothing to the stomach and system. A tasty source of soluble fibre.

Ingredients
- 1 cup water (or herbal tea)
- 2 tablespoons lemon juice
- 5 large apples
- 1 tablespoon ground cinnamon
- ⅓ cup dark brown sugar

Method
Bring the water and lemon juice to the boil in a saucepan. Meanwhile peel, core and quarter the apples. Add the apple chunks and cinnamon to the hot water, cover and simmer for 20 minutes. Add the sugar and, stirring constantly, simmer for a further 5 minutes. Purée with a hand blender or in a food processor. Delicious hot or cold. Keeps for a week in the fridge.

Creamed Banana

Restorative and probiotic.

Method

Blend 1 ripe banana with 50g of natural yoghurt and 1 tablespoon of oats. Serve chilled.

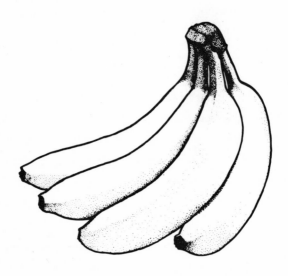

DIGESTIVE COMPLICATIONS

The main culprits in inefficient digestion are indigestion, bloating, trapped wind and flatulence. Other gastric juice and acidity-related issues are heartburn and acid reflux (see page 167). For a dodgy stomach related to food poisoning or gastric flu see page 230, while diarrhoea (see page 95) and constipation (see page 75) also feature as separate entries.

Indigestion/dyspepsia: indigestion is a dysfunction of the digestive system linked to excess stomach acid – presenting as the sensation of fullness after a meal with varying degrees of intensity of discomfort in the upper abdomen. It is sometimes accompanied by heartburn (see page 167), hiccups (see page 171), regurgitation and nausea (see page 204). It can be a precursor to or a symptom of gastroenteritis (see page 230) or a peptic ulcer. It is most commonly thought of as a reaction to spicy food, but in truth any food can cause digestive acids to flare up. Indigestion can also be triggered by alcohol consumption and certain prescription medications, and can be symptomatic of pregnancy or stress.

Garden treatments

Traditionally 'bitters' were utilised as digestants – gentian, dandelion and artichoke being the most popular. Gentian root and dandelion also augment the digestion of proteins and fats. Milk thistle tincture is effective, but simple yarrow tea works just as well. Carminative herbs such as angelica, chamomile, fennel or lemon balm speed up digestion and reduce gas. Peppermint tea is a supreme digestive, accelerating the process and the time it takes the stomach to empty and so cutting short acidic reactions. Lovage root is a digestive. Aloe vera juice is not easy to standardise in the domestic kitchen from home-grown supplies and, while it soothes the digestive tract and stomach, it can be laxative or emetic depending on intensity – a tablespoon of the inner gel blitzed in 8fl oz of water should be sipped to assay intensity. Store-bought is a good option.

Kitchen support

Ginger promotes a digestive-boosting assimilation of food and can also be helpful with the ancillary symptoms of nausea, belching and flatulence. Use with dill, coriander, basil, caraway, cardamom and rosemary to stimulate speedy digestion. While spicy food can exacerbate, some condiments can address discomfort – both black pepper and mustard stimulate the taste buds for extra digesting saliva and signal secretions of digestive hydrochloric acid within the stomach. This does mean more acid but it works to give a quick turnaround – the bloating and ancillary complications are 'un-digestion' complications.

Indigestion can persist beyond a post-meal flare-up and many people find relief with

Yarrow

100

a snack of some grapes (ten or so will hit the spot) or some slices of apple. Both contain phytochemicals that calm digestive upset. Pineapple contains digestive enzymes that can help reduce flare-up. Green tea with some honey is a good way to end a meal and deliver some calming principles to the digestive system.

No Gripes Grape, Apple and Shredded Fennel Salad

Ingredients
- 10 or so grapes
- ½ cup fennel bulb
- 1 apple
- Lemon juice
- Crème fraiche (or other coating/salad dressing)

Method
Halve and chill the grapes. Shred the fennel. Peel, core and dice the apple, then toss it in a dash of lemon juice to slow oxidisation. Combine all the ingredients with a dollop of crème fraiche or sour cream, serve and enjoy.

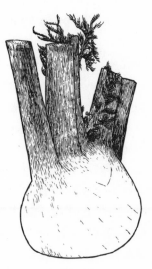

Fennel

Angelica and Lemon Balm Tea

Angelica root is more potent than the leaves but it needs to be properly dried before use. For indigestion purposes, the leaf tea delivers the phytochemical we require and the flavour is pleasant with lemon balm added.

Method

Gather enough foliage of each plant to yield a chopped teaspoon each – add this to a cup of boiling water and infuse for 10 minutes. Leaves can be harvested in greater quantity and dried to make a blend of equal quantity by volume.

Bloating, trapped wind and flatulence are generally related to poor digestion or bad food choices that cause gas build-up in your stomach and intestines.

Bloating: apart from the pressure of fullness, sometimes cramp or abdominal pain can accompany the situation. The most common causes of abdominal bloating include overeating, eating too fast, swallowing air (gulping, chewing gum, etc.), intolerance to dairy products and other food groups, prescription medications, overgrowth of bacteria in the small bowel or intestinal parasites. It can lead to, or be associated with, constipation (see page 75), heartburn (see page 167), belching and weight gain. In some instances, it accompanies menstruation.

Trapped wind is the sensation of needing to burp or fart to alleviate the bloating pressure by gaseous release. It can be an uncomfortable sensation. While there are ways to encourage a gaseous release, and I will include them here, treating digestive sluggishness is the key to both linked conditions. To do so with herbs that are also antibacterial and antimicrobial is beneficial to compromised gut flora.

Flatulence is a by-product of eating. Gases such as hydrogen, methane and carbon dioxide are naturally released during the digestive process and are later expelled either by belching from the mouth or 'breaking wind' from the other end. 'Breaking wind' has some connection to the medical terminology, which comes from the Latin *flatus* – 'blowing, a breaking wind'. It is quite normal to have an average of between ten and twenty wind-expelling occurrences per day (speak for yourself, I hear you say). Problematic or excessive flatulence is generally an issue of poor digestion and the main treatments tackle a sluggish system – but do eat slowly, as gulping air with your food is a major contributor to flatulence. Flatulence can accompany irritable bowel syndrome or food allergies. It can also be symptomatic of bacterial infection in the gut (see page 230).

Garden treatments

Astragalus is full of potent polysaccharides, saponins and flavonoids that boost digestive health and increase the body's metabolic rate to promote a faster and fuller elimination of waste. Peppermint tea is pro-digestive and long utilised to help relieve bloating and abdominal discomfort – all mints act the same way.

Yarrow tea before meals helps inhibit gaseous build-up. Dandelion salad or dandelion root tea is known in gardeners' lore as a remedy for bloating and digestive complaints, alongside its colloquial name of 'piss in the bed', highlighting its diuretic value. It is one of the few diuretics that don't deplete potassium from the system – in fact it adds it, which is key to stopping bloating occurring (more on that in the 'Kitchen support' section opposite). It also supplies a good mix of magnesium, calcium and iron as well as vitamins A, B-complex, C and D – all helping to control stress levels which can contribute to or exacerbate digestive ailments.

For **bloating and trapped wind**, herbalists and naturopaths would suggest carminative herbs with compounds that promote the expulsion of trapped gas. The mints (spear, pepper and common) fit into this group, as do half the culinary herbs we use – it's the reason they are employed: the flavour preference came later in our cultural evolution. So add dill, fennel, basil, parsley, oregano, caraway or cumin to meals, or take as herbal tea. Chamomile tea is both calming and carminative, and can address bacterial infection.

For **flatulence**, in western medical systems peppermint tea is long established as a reliever of flatulence and gastrointestinal problems, but we don't have to rely on just one herb. In fact we have two good routes to choose from. First, we can select carminative herbs which prevent gaseous build-up and help facilitate the expulsion of what has accumulated. Second, we can opt for digestive herbs to promote fuller digestion and absorption – with increased gastrointestinal efficiency the issue of excess gas is lessened. Carminative herbs from the garden include angelica (both leaf and root), basil, catmint, chamomile, echinacea, fennel, goldenrod, lemon balm, lovage, mint, motherwort and nigella. Common garden-grown digestive herbs (note some overlap with carminative properties) include catmint, chamomile, echinacea, lemon balm, slippery elm bark and yarrow.

Kitchen support

Both antibacterial garlic and probiotic live yoghurt can aid the healthy functioning of the digestive system. A tablespoon of apple cider vinegar in a small glass of water or herbal tea before meals can kick-start the digestive processes and relieve gas build-up. Remember, before you begin to cook or serve, that this problem is often about eating too fast, too much in one sitting, or too overly processed foods. An excess of salt in our diets can push our potassium levels off kilter and have knock-on effects for general health – potassium is key to digestion. Our digestive tract is lined with smooth muscle tissue that contracts and releases under the signalling of electrolytes – particularly potassium – to move food through the stages of digestion, nutrient absorption and waste elimination. Eating more potassium-rich foods (avocados, asparagus, dark leafy greens, tomatoes, potatoes, peas and beans, citrus fruits, melons and of course bananas) will enhance what is known as 'intestinal motility' (the motions) and decrease gastrointestinal discomfort.

In terms of menstrual bloating, aromatherapy has a pleasant solution: a blend of lemon balm and geranium massaged around the stomach and abdomen in a clockwise direction.

Foot on the Gas Fennel and Mint Tea

A stimulating anise-flavoured tea to prompt digestive function and settle the stomach.

Method

Simply infuse 1 teaspoon of fennel seeds and 1 teaspoon of any variety of mint into a pint of boiling water. Steep for 7–10 minutes and thereafter sip freely. Sweeten with honey if desired.

Trapped Wind Asanas

Asanas are yoga poses and who hasn't attempted a yoga move and felt a free movement of gas? Even a simple squat or a bend over to straighten the mat can do the trick. OK, you're bloated, so I'm not going to get you to put your foot on your forehead, but maybe it's time to do some pretend garden Pilates or outside yoga. You can do it in the house but why not enjoy the daylight? A little physicality always helps but this pose/exercise should release the pressure.

Method

Lie flat on your back and slowly pull your feet back towards your bum – legs bent at the knees but feet flat on the floor. Hold the pose for a few minutes. You can gently rub your stomach but this position naturally facilitates air to move in the right direction.

If that fails, pull your knees towards your chest and hold for a moment.

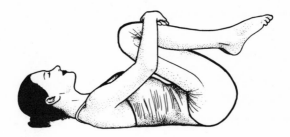

EAR AILMENTS

Ear ailments are not just for children. I have divided them into ache, infection, wax build-up and tinnitus, which cover the prime afflictions of adults and children.

Ear ache can affect one or both ears, manifest as a constant sharp pain, a hot sensation or dull throb, or it can be more of a come-and-go experience. Ear ache affects children much more frequently than adults – in fact it is one of the most common reasons parents visit a GP or avail of an out-of-hours service with their child, the other being fever (see page 133). All the treatments here are child friendly.

There are many common causes of ear ache – infection and wax build-up are the most common, but trapped water (swimmer's ear) or fluid build-up (glue ear) are also high on the list. On occasion, a boil, eczema (see page 84), a throat infection (see page 223) or tonsillitis (see page 228) can refer pain to the area. Likewise, referred pain can come from trigeminal neuralgia (see page 208) or a dental abscess (see page 242). Sometimes it can be caused by an injury from a cotton bud or other object used to clear or scratch an itchy ear canal. Perforated eardrums require a GP visit.

Top tip

Blow off the pain. Adults can use this method but it is also great for children. Blowing is a distraction method that brings the focus of the brain away from pain perception and onto the task. Blowing also activates jaw muscles and ear movements that can clear blockages and stimulate blood flow to the ear – bringing the body's own healing mechanisms into play. Make a paper windmill or a pinwheel and play the blowing game with your child – depending on their age, pretending to blow out the candles on teddy's birthday cake or blowing bubbles. Making fish faces and boop-blop noises or steam-train noises help too.

Ear infection: both bacteria and viruses can cause ear infections. Infections of the ear canal are known clinically as *otitis externa*, while infections of the eardrum or the middle ear are known as *otitis media*. No matter the location, the symptoms can include pain or pressure, tinnitus (see page 112), loss of hearing (mostly temporary), discharge from the ear and, because the ear is implicated in our spatial perception and physical balance, the sensation of travel sickness or vertigo.

Ear wax: over-the-counter treatments for ear wax fill shelves in pharmacies and even find their way into supermarkets. Ear wax is a natural phenomenon, also known as cerumen – this yellowish waxy substance is regularly secreted within the ear canal as part of the ear's cleaning and lubrication mechanism. It also helps protect the ear canal from bacteria, fungi and water. Problems arise when cerumen builds up and solidifies into a wax plug, causing swelling, pain and decreased efficiency of hearing. It often resolves on its own, as talking and movements of the jaw can dislodge and keep wax moving. Reading this page aloud or singing your favourite song might work too – but softening the wax will aid natural clearance and the remedies below will help with that. In some instances a GP will syringe ears if the build-up is too large to shift or too painful to wait for nature.

Garden treatments

Yarrow, mullein and lavender are traditional remedies for ear infection, used as an infusion to make rinses or a gauze pad compress. They can also be infused in olive oil and used as clearing drops to remove wax and debris and deliver some antiseptic and analgesic relief. Chamomile, goldenrod and St John's wort all have anti-inflammatory action when used in ear oils, but the supreme remedy is antimicrobial and cleansing garlic, home-grown or straight from the supermarket – peel, crush and simply infuse in olive oil overnight.

Kitchen support

Olive oil is soothing and cleansing as drops in its own right and makes an excellent carrier for antiseptic and anti-inflammatory herbs. It is also a perfect way of bringing the antiviral and antibacterial action of garlic into play. Some raw garlic juice mixed with a little oil can be placed in the ear as one would with over-the-counter drops. Sipping green tea is an infection buster as it boosts the curing capacity of gamma delta T cells in any infection. Stepping up your immune system is great for hard-to-reach infections, such as in the ear. Foods that boost the immune system include mushrooms – from button and shiitake to the medicinal reishi mushroom – which encourage the production of white blood cells. Natural yoghurt is a catalyst for your gut-supported immune system and any food rich in zinc or vitamin C will also give it a boost. When it comes to wax, simply eating something can have an effect. Doesn't matter what. Healthy or a wicked treat? Just eat. The actions of a chewing jaw vibrate in the ear and this helps remove excess wax.

Garlic Ear Oil

For aches, infections and wax removal. There are two ways to obtain this:

1. The traditional way is to peel and smash all of the cloves in a head of garlic, add to a jam jar or 250ml bottle filled with olive oil and allow it to sun infuse over a two-week period. The resulting oil is great as a culinary drizzle and you will have it in store for the next ache or wax build-up.

2. The second way – in case of urgency – is a quick blitz method. Simply add peeled garlic cloves to a blender with 250ml of olive oil. Blitz and decant to a jar resting in boiling water or to a bain-marie – allow it to warm and rest in the heat for 30 minutes, swirling up the bits with a wooden spoon from time to time. Finally, let sedimentation happen naturally and strain off some

infused oil to use. It can continue to infuse on a windowsill and you can stir, let settle and syphon off some oil each day until the infection or wax is remedied. This lasts for several months to a year, as the garlic is antimicrobial.

How to use the ear oil effectively

As long as the ear drum is not ruptured, you can put a few drops of oil into the ear channel/canal. You can use it at room temperature, but warm oil is more soothing and breaks wax down quicker. Infused oil can be stored in any bottle or jar with a lid or dropper. Before use, you can bring it above room temperature by placing the bottle in a pan of warm water for several minutes. Do check the suitability of the oil temperature on your wrist. Lean your head over the sink and drop or pour in a little oil. Insert a little cotton wool to hold in the oil and warmth – if necessary repeat the treatment in the other ear. After 15 minutes you can remove the cotton wool – have some extra cotton wool or tissue handy as excess oil or wax may run out of the ear. Repeat applications, several times a day over a few days, should resolve the issue.

Tinnitus is the condition of ringing, buzzing or other auditory sensations in the ears, most often triggered by exposure to loud noise or a side effect of ear-wax (see page 109) blockage. However, it can manifest as a prolonged or recurring experience due to age-related hearing loss, an injury to the ear or a circulatory disorder. Tinnitus is present in as much as 90 per cent of people suffering from the metabolic condition known as hyperinsulinemia (increased levels of insulin in the bloodstream), one of the precursors to type 2 diabetes.

Garden treatments

A tincture of black cohosh or gingko tea can be employed as a circulatory tonic beneficial for tinnitus. Hawthorn is also great at boosting peripheral circulation. Feverfew and meadowsweet have applications in pain relief and sensitising issues. To relieve pressure, remove wax and treat ear infections contributing to ringing by putting a few drops of olive oil into the ear canal. The oil can be boosted by infusion with ear herbs – mullein, garlic and mint are the traditional recommendations, but lavender, geranium and calendula are also suitable.

I mention gamma-linolenic acid (GLA) a lot in this book. Amongst other things it is metabolised in the body to form dihomo-gamma-linolenic acid (DGLA), a vital component in the production of prostaglandin E1. That's the hormone-like chemical active in immune-system response, inflammation control and stable blood pressure – all actions helpful to tinnitus. DGLA also prevents platelets from sticking together, improves blood flow and strengthens blood vessel tone – even more good news for tinnitus. The highest source of GLA is borage oil, followed by

Geranium

113

blackcurrant oil and then evening primrose oil. Borage oil can be up to five times more potent than evening primrose oil. The issue with borage oil is that cold-pressed home-produced oils can contain amabiline and other unsaturated pyrrolizidine alkaloids, which are not good for the liver at all – but store-bought oil is standardised and safe.

Kitchen support

Ginger can address the dizziness that sometimes accompanies tinnitus and also improves natural defences against the underlying conditions that contribute to ringing in the ears. Sesame seeds have a long history of use in traditional Chinese medicine to address tinnitus. Reducing salt intake can help. Excess salt increases blood pressure and restricts blood vessels – including in the ear canal. Avoid monosodium glutamate (MSG), which metabolises in the body to become an excitatory neuro-transmitter. It triggers neurons to keep firing until they deplete and die off – including neurons that line and facilitate the auditory pathway. Other flavour enhancers, notably artificial sweeteners, can act likewise. Cut out the saturated and trans-fats that reduce blood flow and opt for unsaturated fats (vegetable, nut and fish sources), which can help increase blood flow and lower blood pressure. Omega-3 fatty acids reduce inflammation and diminish pain perception.

Black Cohosh Root Tea

The roots contain vitamins A, B1, B2, B3, C and K, calcium, iron, magnesium, potassium, sodium, zinc and salicylic acid – beneficial in both immune and inflammation responses. Dried root is traditional but fresh root can also be used.

Method

Clean and slice the roots and leave to dry for over a week (with an optimum drying temperature of 36–38°C) in a shaded, aired location, or clean the fresh root well and slice to use straight away. Boiling water that has cooled for 2 minutes is best to make the tea. Allow a few minutes to infuse. This tea is traditionally sipped cool.

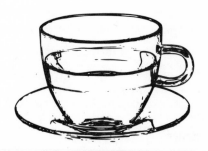

EYE AILMENTS

We gardeners live through our eyes – making a garden is a visual creation as well as a physical construction. So eyesight is vital. We make a garden not just to harvest from or potter about in but also to look at – to be seen. But we are often in the glare of the sun, staring at caterpillar holes in favourite plants, squinting at the seed tray for signs of movement – and let's not forget rubbing our eyes in disbelief at the prices in garden centres. For the consequences of all that, help is at hand.

EYESTRAIN AND TIRED EYES

We all have tired-eye days but if you're having a tired-eye week then you need to get proactive. Strained eyes can be soothed physically by bathing with cooled herbal tisanes but you will need to tackle the underlying causes – do you need glasses, less time on social media, larger print at the library, etc.? Or is a nutritional deficiency or an underlying medical condition affecting your eyesight? Always visit an optician or GP if you have any vision irregularities.

Garden treatments

Strained eyes can be bathed or rinsed with fennel tea or a decoction of eyebright to soothe the eye and ease some physical symptoms. Consuming some edible petals and colourful berries may help strengthen the mechanisms of focus and light/dark adaption, thus reducing stress and strain. My personal favourite would be calendulas, which not only are edible in salads but also make great infusions and deliver lutein. This plays a particular role in reducing the risk of age-related macular degeneration by providing a yellow-orange pigment (macular pigment) that protects the macula from the blue light spectrum and any potential damaging photo-oxidative effects. Rustle up a healthy alfresco lunch – beyond the leafy greens – and enjoy raspberries, oranges, peaches, cherries, bilberries and blueberries for extra lutein top-ups.

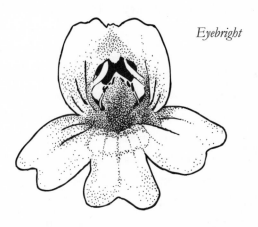

Eyebright

Kitchen support

Carotenoids are the colourful pigments in our fruits and vegetables. They are beneficial to health in general but are well known or frequently promoted as precursors to vitamin A. However, not all carotenoids convert to vitamin A. For example the red pigment of watermelon and tomatoes known as lycopene does not. So if you are drawn to picking colourful food, aim for the bright-orange spectrum – packed with beta-carotene, which yields more vitamin A than alpha- or gamma-carotene in the other ranges of the spectrum. Vitamin A is vital for healthy vision and vegetables with lutein (kale, spinach, broccoli and other dark leafy veg) and other helpful carotenoids (carrots, mango, watermelon, sweet potato, bell peppers, tomatoes) will supply that and help to strengthen the retina and eye tissue.

Daisy Water

The common lawn daisy derives its name from 'day's eye', a hint that the flowers close at night, but it also has a history as an ophthalmic herb. The flowers contain tannin and the foliage traces of calcium and magnesium. Distilled daisy water is long recorded as being sipped for failing eyesight and inflammations of the eye, while as a rinse daisy water is soothing to strained and tired eyes. Distilled daisy water can be made by the hydrosol method using one-third of a cup of flower heads to a cup of water. If distillation is too laborious for you then a tisane of daisy flowers and leaf – 1 tablespoon herb to 1 cup boiling water – is a quick version. Let it cool for an hour before straining and using. It's best used the same day but can be stored in the fridge for a few days.

Daisy

Cucumber Eye Reviver for Tired Eyes

Cucumbers have a high water content and so they chill well. The combination of the moisture and coolness of a chilled cucumber slice will help soothe eyes, sockets and surrounding skin. Cucumbers have just the right trace amounts of salt to draw excess water and toxins from the facial tissue surrounding the eyes, reducing puffiness and, cosmetically, simultaneously toning and firming the sockets, lids and skin around the eyes.

Method
Chill a cucumber, slice into circular pads to place over the eyes for 5–15 minutes – slice thinly and, rather than having two thick goggles, apply several thin layers to better mould to the contours of your eyes and face.

CONJUNCTIVITIS AND STYES
The two most common eye complaints after strain are conjunctivitis and styes – one affects the eye, the other the eyelid. The treatments here address both.

Conjunctivitis: presenting as redness and dryness, and often with a discharge of sticky fluid, conjunctivitis is an inflammation of the conjunctiva – the membrane that covers the entirety of your eyeball and the inside of your eyelids. Conjunctivitis can be bacterial or viral – either way it is quite contagious and easily passed from one eye to another, let alone from person to person. You may also experience burning, blurred vision and eye pain. Your GP may advise prescription drops, but if you wish to try natural remedies or use them in support of conventional treatments then you can't go wrong with the herbal tisanes listed below to bathe or rinse the eyes.

A **stye** is a bacterial infection – not of the eye as such but of an eyelash follicle – or an inflammation of one or more of the sebaceous glands within your eyelid. It can be sore, cause blurriness or just be unsightly with crusting and weeping. Like conjunctivitis, styes can be contagious and transmit quickly from eye to eye.

Garden treatments

Many garden herbs are suitable for eyebaths – fennel, chamomile, lawn daisy, goldenseal and eyebright all have a potent and long history as treatments for conjunctivitis. The caffeic acid in both eyebright and goldenseal acts as an antiseptic, while the others all have cleansing and soothing attributes. Cooled infusions of any of these herbs can be used to make compresses, and actual poultices of elderflower, eyebright and chickweed are also beneficial to eye health. Castor oil as a topical skin 'gel' contains ricinoleic acid, which is strongly anti-inflammatory and analgesic.

Kitchen support

Tea bag compresses are often the first port of call, with tannins to shrink swelling and clean away hardened discharge. Cooled tea (black or green) rinses will soften crusting and heal causative factors. By way of dietary support, crunching on carrots, apples or celery will help get the antihistamine levels up and the irritation down, and any of the immune system foods (see page 65) will be beneficial too.

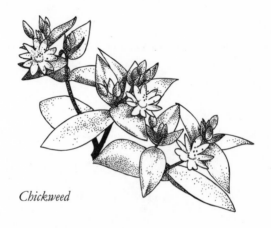

Chickweed

Black Tea Compress

The heat is remedial but the tannic acid is also helpful to lessen inflammation and tackle infection. If the eye is very sticky or encrusted, cooled tea on a cotton pad can help cleanse.

Method

Make a cup of black tea with a tea bag. Remove the tea bag and allow to sit on a saucer to cool for a moment. Squeeze off excess tea and utilise as a warm compress.

Fennel and Chamomile Eyebath

Both these herbs have the capacity to heal and soothe the conjunctiva and are traditionally used to cleanse eyes and reduce itching and inflammation.

Method

Put a tablespoon of each in a cup of boiling water. You know the drill – let it cool and use the liquid as a rinse or drops.

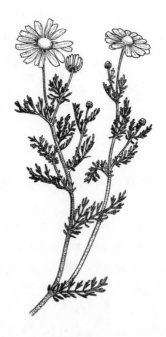

Chamomile

FATIGUE

We all get tired from time to time, but sometimes tiredness is less of a hint from the body that it's bedtime, or a 'cease and desist' on that total dig-over of the allotment, and more a case of either periodic or chronic fatigue.

GENERAL FATIGUE

Tiredness: when not due to overwork, under-sleep or poor nutrition (not enough food for energy release, energy-sapping food or a diet lacking B vitamins), this can be related to impaired thyroid function. A GP can test for that and dietary changes can sort it out. In some instances over-active adrenals can trigger crashes and the garden can sort that out. Occasionally tiredness is not just a time of low energy midway through the day or before bedtime, but is a form of periodic fatigue.

Periodic fatigue is prolonged tiredness due to illness recovery, situational depression, stress, physical overexertion, malnourishment or a combination of these. It generally resolves with bed rest, decreased workload, dietary change and a sense of rejuvenation. It is not a complex illness, such as chronic fatigue, and resolves within days of you taking care of yourself.

Garden treatments

Sometimes a little fresh air and garden aromas can clear the mind, bring about a relaxation response and set you up for a good day or a good night's sleep. For aroma, rosemary is rejuvenating for concentration and diminishing of tiredness. Lavender is adaptogenic – it helps the body cope better with stress. Take as a tea or aromatherapeutically, or have a lavender bath made from a few drops of essential oil or plant parts. Chamomile tea soothes nerves and tensions and calms the system. Some herbalists prescribe valerian and plants that promote sleep as way to eradicate tiredness – that's certainly better than trying to pump up your energy and adrenals with sugary foods and caffeine.

See more about sleep on page 178 but think too about waking hours and what depletes you during that time. Do less of what drains you. That may mean taking your lunch away from dreary canteens and drearier colleagues and getting a burst of daylight or change of scenery. Or it may be going for a walk after work before the rush-hour commute to skip that stress. We get adrenal spikes from stress – it's the evolutionary 'fight or flight', which meant you ran from the tiger or fought the tiger. You can do neither to the traffic light. Aim for a better quality of life. Spending more time in nature is rewarding and energising.

Herbal teas recommended for short-term fatigue include bee balm, passionflower, mint, rosemary, chamomile and gingko. Ginkgo increases the production of adenosine triphosphate (ATP), which helps with cellular metabolism of energy and is also involved in how the brain metabolises glucose for its energy. Think too of adaptogens (which help the body adapt to stresses and return to normal settings) such as liquorice root (its glycyrrhizin content enhances the activation of cortisol and stress control) or Siberian ginseng, which actively supports adrenal function and promotes stamina.

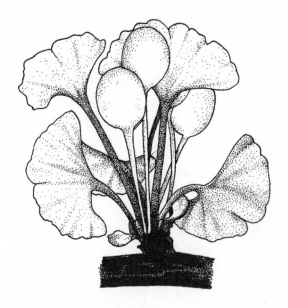

Ginkgo

Kitchen support

To fight your fatigue you need to avoid the sugar crash, the roller-coaster caffeine ride and other similar stimulants, and instead choose foods that release energy slowly and keep you topped up for sustained periods. Sustained energy foods include oatmeal, quinoa, whole grains, beans and proteins. More fruit and veg is recommended to energise, detox and support the body's general health – but not all fruits and veg are equal when it comes to relieving tiredness or releasing prolonged energy. In terms of fruits, apples, pears, plums, melons, cherries and berries are good – slow release, valuable fibre and nice phytochemicals too. Remember juices, dried fruits and canned fruits are all quick-release and sugar spiking. With veg it's all about the non-starchy options to maintain a slow release of their carbohydrates and balance the starchy ones on the plate – so choose broccoli, cauliflower, spinach, kale and asparagus – the iron in these also remedies fatigue.

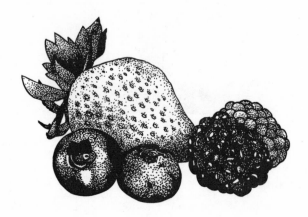

Energy Breakfast Muesli

Fast- and slow-release energy to keep you going throughout the day.

Ingredients

- 120g rolled oats
- 40g rye flakes
- 10g bran
- 25g flaked almonds
- 25g hazelnut nibs
- 25g raisins or sultanas
- 25g dried apple pieces – diced
- 15g roughly chopped dried apricots (or dried figs)

Method

You can toast the grains and nuts at 160°C (325°F/Gas Mark 3) for 8–10 minutes or use them untreated. If toasting, cool completely before adding the dried fruits and stirring them through. This stores well in an airtight container. Serve with milk, natural yoghurt or cream and a sliced banana or strawberries or even a sprinkle of blueberries.

Original Muesli

Once upon a time muesli was cutting-edge nutritional medicine, developed by Swiss physician Maximilian Bircher-Benner around 1900 to treat jaundice and fatigue. This is the original recipe – one that was not a collection of dry ingredients as we find on supermarket shelves today or the version on the previous page, but instead with an emphasis on raw fruit and oat soaking.

Ingredients
- 1 tablespoon rolled oats
- 1 tablespoon lemon juice
- 1 tablespoon chopped nuts – preferably almonds and/or hazelnuts
- 1–2 tablespoons milk or cream
- 1 small apple

Method
Soak the oats overnight in 2 tablespoons of water. Next day add the lemon juice and chopped nuts and fold together, pour on the milk or cream and grate some apple over the mix before serving.

CHRONIC FATIGUE

Chronic fatigue syndrome is not just tiredness: it is a complex and chronic illness manifesting as, amongst other symptoms, a sustained tiredness (diagnosed after a prolonged experience of five to six months) that cannot be remedied with a bout of bed rest. Ancillary symptoms include muscle and joint pain, headaches (see page 149), poor digestion (see page 99), poor concentration capacity, irritability and sometimes confusion and memory issues. Dehydration, low blood pressure, anxiety/depression and insomnia (see page 178) may also feature.

A single cause has not been discovered – many believe it to be bacterial or viral, or a residual complex of a previous viral infection (including human Epstein-Barr, rubella, herpes virus 6 and human retroviruses). But it can also relate to immune system impairment, hypotension or hormonal issues – some case histories reveal persistent candida infections (see page 53). Alongside the advice given here, do avail of the antiviral and antibacterial herbs and foods mentioned throughout this book.

Garden treatments

One of the big problems is that sleep becomes non-refreshing, but a few drops of lavender essential oil on the pillow or some cut lavender bundles inside the pillowcase or hung above the bed can reset the limbic region of the brain and promote better sleep. The second concern is that a system under the strain of fatigue becomes inefficient and so the consideration of metabolic foods and herbs becomes helpful.

Let the garden be your temple for 20 minutes each day. Tai

chi, yoga or movement meditations not only energise the body (mind and spirit), but also provide a relaxation response and release from fatigue. I know you may be too tired to make a cup of tea sometimes but, honestly, even if today you just stand in the garden and pretend for 30 seconds that you are (in slow motion) directing a fighter plane, waving to a passing ship or breast-stroking across a warm pool you will reap the reward. The gift is that the energy of movement, the fresh air in the lungs, the contribution of daylight to circadian rhythms and sunlight to vitamin D levels are boosting you towards recovery. Try 35 seconds tomorrow.

Kitchen support

Diet is important with all health issues, but here it is deeply significant. Leaving aside food as medicine for a moment: foods are either energy givers or energy sappers. What you eat is important to provide for, and not deplete, your energy reserves. Takeaways and processed foods can stress the adrenal glands, whatever about adding sluggishness. Sugars, white flour and salt can deplete nutrients and crash the metabolism for periods. Make fresh fruit and vegetables a priority to detox your body and bring energy levels up. Then you can think of the ones that work medicinally – foods for mood, those that are antibacterial, immune boosters, etc. (skim the *Kitchen supports* section of the ancillary symptoms already mentioned to find more options).

Ginger, garlic and honey all boost the immune system, are antibacterial and help with post-viral recovery too. But top of my list are mushrooms as potent sources of vitamin D (which supports mood and a sense of well-being), immune stimulants and nutrition. In particular there is a group of what has become known as the medicinal mushrooms – maitake, shiitake and reishi – sometimes available on supermarket shelves if you don't have a local Asian market, but also available in capsule form in your nearest health shop. If you can get fresh do – you can cook with them as you would any edible mushroom.

Suimono-Style Mushroom Broth

Because I am using what used to be known as Japanese mushrooms, I thought it would be nice to go for a *Suimono,* a traditional Japanese broth or 'food you can sip' – or at least my speedy take on it.

Ingredients
- 100g chopped fresh or dried maitake, shiitake or reishi mushrooms
- 100g silken tofu
- 3–4 cups water
- 1 teaspoon dashi stock or miso paste
- 2 scallions
- 1 teaspoon soy sauce

Method
Clean the mushrooms and cut into thin lengths. Rinse and dice the tofu into nice square chunks. Bring the water to a boil and

add the mushrooms, dashi stock and tofu. Bring back to the boil, then simmer for 5 minutes. Slice the scallions into coins, add to the broth and simmer for a further 2–3 minutes. Remove from the heat, add the soy sauce and serve. Pepper and salt to taste are optional.

FEVER

Not always a lovely way to burn, fever signifies an underlying medical condition – often an infection – that may need the expertise of a medical professional. For babies and infants even a slight elevation of core temperature needs attention, while for adults the general rule is that temperatures above 38.9°C (102°F) are perilous. The normal or standard adult temperature is a fluctuating affair and can vary from body to body but a guide is around 37°C (98.6°F). That said, fever is part of the body's own healing response to kill off invading organisms such as bacteria or viral infections that thrive at normal body temperature. There is a case to be made to let a fever run its course – sweating is the thermostat control to keep us safe in the process – but sustained, high or childhood fevers are a concern and medical advice is best sought quickly.

Garden treatments

Feverfew gets its name from the Latin *febrifugia*, which means 'to drive out fevers'. Herbalists have used it since the Greek physician Dioscorides recommended it back in the first century. While it is great to drive away headaches and drive down inflammation, I am not fully convinced of its ability to chemically lessen a high temperature. It does show some antimicrobial action and the clue to its success is in that, perhaps, more than in assumed refrigerant properties.

There is a whole group of herbs – the febrifuges, aka the

anti-pyretics – that diminish fever. They include linden leaf, mint, meadowsweet, yarrow, hyssop, chamomile, catmint and borage. Rather than choosing herbs to suppress a fever, I reach for a cooling device, be that a fan or hairdryer on cool, or a damp chilled towel on the forehead. These instantly help with how we moderate and experience the heat. I do, however, like the twin approach of ending a fever by tackling its causes while also cooling down – so the treatments and supports here involve internal antimicrobial action. Anti-infection and immune-stimulant herbs include elderberry, echinacea, thyme, yarrow, gingko and lemon balm. Fuchsia berries are said to reduce fevers – they are edible and great in a compote or fruit salad.

Kitchen support

An old folk remedy for fever reduction was to crush a few cloves of garlic to a paste and apply it to the chest or feet. Certainly internal consumption of garlic can help lower a fever by boosting the body's immune system to better fight the underlying infection. Garlic is also toxic to many bacterial and viral strains that trigger fever. Antimicrobial and immune system boosters include ginger, oregano, turmeric, cinnamon, clove and honey.

You may have heard the old saying 'feed a cold, starve a fever' – well it's half right. It was based upon the assumption that eating heated the body – hence eat for a cold – and not eating might just let the body cool – hence starve the fever. One thing I remember fondly from my Christian Brothers schooling was the saying and spelling aide-memoire 'to assume is to make an ass of u and me'. So half right, I said – in fact it's good to feed a cold but it's also good to feed a fever. I'm not even necessarily talking about medicinal food (but I am too), as a raised temperature increases metabolism and expends more calories and depletes energy reserves – so eat to replenish. Even more important than eating is drinking fluids to offset dehydration.

Lemon, Lime and Linden Iced Tea

Cooling and remedial.

Method
Make a pot of linden tea. Add the juice of one lime and the juice of one lemon. Chill in the fridge and sip throughout the day. The linden is anti-pyretic and somewhat sedative and the juices add extra flavour and plenty of vitamin C.

Wellness Spread

Excellent on toast or the bread of your choice to keep energy up and tackle infections.

Method
Stir 1 tablespoon of turmeric, 1 tablespoon of cinnamon and half a teaspoon of ground cloves into 150g honey.

GUM HEALTH

Bleeding gums can signal gum disease or recent tartar build-up. Sometimes improper technique or over-exertion with the floss or the brush can traumatise the gum tissue and lead to bleeding or inflammation. Some oral bleeding can relate to deficiencies in vitamin K or flag a more serious platelet disorder – so if it's not resolving quickly see your dentist or GP.

Garden treatments

Hawthorn berries and bilberry fruits strengthen gum tissue. A spit-rinse of horsetail tea can, through its cleansing action and silica content, actually fortify the connective tissues of the mouth and gums. Tincture or tisane rinses of selfheal, tormentil and field scabious are remedial. Sipping sage, lavender, yarrow or chamomile tea will coat the gum line with natural antiseptic and decrease bacterial levels.

Kitchen support

Rinsing with salt water is helpful – boosting that saline solution with the power of thyme, lavender, rosemary, chamomile or yarrow will promote gum healing through suppression of inflammation and bacteria, and via sterilisation of any wound.

Horsetail and Yarrow Gargle

Haemostatic, disinfecting and anti-inflammatory, yarrow is the herb of the Greek warrior Achilles, who used it to stop bleeding and disinfect wounds. Horsetail tones gums and soothes inflammation. The inclusion of a little salt also cleans and disinfects further.

Method

Simply make an infusion of 1 teaspoon of salt and 2 teaspoons of each herb to half a cup of boiling water and steep for half an hour. This stores for a week in the fridge. Horsetail tea from a health shop is a good substitute for the fresh herb. Likewise with yarrow.

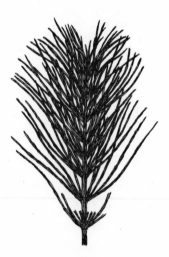

Horsetail

Inflamed gums/gingivitis: inflammation may be caused by underlying tooth decay but mostly it is due to inadequate plaque removal from teeth at the gum line. Plaque can be removed by regular brushing but avoid alcohol-containing mouthwashes, as they can aggravate inflammation. Try instead any of the homemade washes and rinses in this section.

Garden treatments

Aloe vera can cool down inflamed gums and eliminate the bacteria build-up responsible for gingivitis. Simply massage a little sap into the gums. Horsetail tea is restorative to gums. Both yarrow and chamomile tea will coat the gum line with natural antiseptic and decrease bacteria levels.

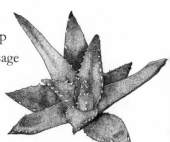

Aloe Vera

Kitchen support

Deficiency in vitamin C can inflame the mouth and gums. Have some citrus juice and include seasonal berries and fruits in your breakfast and lunch not only to top up vitamin C but also to generate an inhospitable environment for bacteria growth. From the spice rack, sage, ginger, cayenne, turmeric and cloves are all anti-inflammatory. For a pinch of antibacterial action try rosemary, mint, coriander/cilantro, basil, nutmeg or garlic.

Simple Salt-Paste Soda Gum Rub

Baking soda is not only a cleanser of plaque and tartar along the gum line, but is anti-inflammatory in its own right.

Method
Simply mix a teaspoon each of baking soda and salt with enough water – a drop at a time – to make a paste, rub along the gums and allow to rest there for 2–3 minutes or as a pre-treatment before brushing. Rinse out with lukewarm water.

Receding gums/gingival recession: receding gums mean that the roots of your teeth become exposed, causing a greater risk of decay and tooth loss, and sensitivity to hot and cold and to some food acids. Heredity can play a part but often it is a case of lacklustre oral hygiene practices (infrequent brushing) or over enthusiasm for a white smile, as too much oral product or brushing too vigorously at the gum line can cause recession. Hormonal changes can impact female gums – fluctuations at puberty, pregnancy and also during menopause can make gums more sensitive and susceptible to gum recession.

Garden treatments
Gingko tea will improve blood circulation to the gums. Teasel root is a traditional gum treatment in Chinese botanical medicine to heal damaged connective or structural tissue. The anti-inflammatory and antibacterial sap of aloe makes a good gum

rub and even a useful toothpaste. Chamomile and yarrow tea can help with oral hygiene.

Kitchen support

Eat your five a day – fruits and vegetables contain many nutrients that maintain gum health. Those rich in vitamin C reduce inflammation and prompt gum regeneration. Many herbal teas, especially the mint family and the antibacterial chamomile, rosemary and sage, are beneficial in addressing any gum diseases triggering recession or resulting from recession. You could also use your pantry supply of coconut oil or sesame oil to try some Ayurveda-style oral health with a mouth-rinse technique called oil pulling. Sip a tablespoon of oil, swish then suck the oil through your teeth for a minute or so, spit and rinse. This strengthens gums, detoxes the mouth, cleans the tongue, removes debris from the teeth, is anodyne and somewhat antiseptic. It works best if you keep it up daily or even twice daily for a few weeks in a row.

Gingko and Ginger Anti-Gingival Tea

These phytochemicals will strengthen gum circulation, remove bacteria and support gum regeneration. This tea can be cooled and stored in the fridge for a week to be used as a daily mouthwash.

Method

Add 5 gingko leaves and 1 teaspoon of chopped ginger root to a cup of boiling water. Allow to rest until cool enough to sip as a beverage, strain away solids and drink at your leisure.

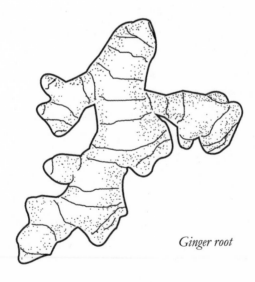

Ginger root

HAEMORRHOIDS/PILES

Haemorrhoids are swollen veins quite similar to varicose veins (see page 250), which may stay internal to or protrude slightly from the anus. There is a slight medical distinction between internal and external, but the treatments here effectively tackle both. Haemorrhoids are a natural part of ageing and often of pregnancy but that does not mean you have to accept the discomfort. If you are young and not pregnant, or young and male then those piles mean you are (forgive the pun) possibly piling on the kilos and/or lacking exercise. Haemorrhoids are also symptomatic of chronic constipation (see page 75) or a congested liver. Piles may bleed, burn, itch and cause pain.

Garden treatments

Once the most popular herbal treatment was a poultice of pilewort, but today perhaps an internal tincture and external compress of horse chestnut extract (see page 252) is the superior vein tonic. Douches or cotton-pad dabs of decoctions of yarrow, lady's mantle or goldenseal root are also remedial. Topically, aloe vera gel is soothing and mildly analgesic, and witch hazel extract is astringent. Consumption of decoctions or tisanes of yellow dock root and dandelion root deliver detox bitters, while rosemary and gingko improve circulation and can help the body resolve or diminish such issues naturally.

Kitchen support

Explore more options to add extra dietary fibre to your daily meals. Excellent sources of fibre include apples, oats, flaxseed, peas, beans, barley and berries. Consume more vibrant-coloured fruits and vegetables, as the bioflavonoids that supply their colour can strengthen the walls of human blood vessels. Phytoconstituents digested from parsley and red grape vine leaves are beneficial to support venal integrity. Apple cider vinegar is a good topical treatment.

Yarrow and Apple Cider Douche

A douche of apple cider vinegar can strengthen capillaries, shrink protrusions, arrest bleeding and address pain. Yarrow is styptic and anti-inflammatory.

Method

Dilute apple cider vinegar in a ratio of 50/50 with haemostatic yarrow tea as a douche, or infuse yarrow foliage in the vinegar for increased potency.

Horse Chestnut and Apple Cider Solution

The tonic action of the horse chestnut complements the astringent properties of the vinegar. In essence, we are making a mother tincture but extracting with apple cider vinegar rather than alcohol.

Method

Harvest a cupful of horse chestnuts, crack the shells and add the inner flesh to half a cup of apple cider vinegar – decant to a storage bottle and leave in a dark cupboard for three weeks. Thereafter remove the solids. The resulting infused vinegar can be diluted 75/25 with water and utilised as a douche, or you can use the solution to make lotions and creams.

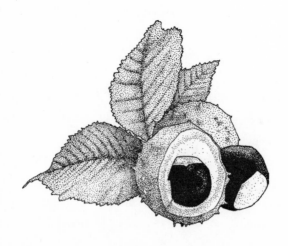

Horse chestnut

HAY FEVER
AND POLLEN ALLERGIES

Some years pollen counts can be particularly high and even non-hay-fever sufferers find themselves overwhelmed and experiencing hay-fever symptoms, including sneezing, a runny nose and watery or itchy eyes. Some adults may have one or two reactions but do not develop repeat hay-fever attacks. Childhood hay fever often lessens in intensity with age and may even disappear altogether. Some asthmatics are more prone to pollen than dust or other triggers, so this section could also be beneficial to help control asthma attacks.

Hay fever is often seen as a seasonal allergy triggered by microscopic pollen grains. Those grains are protein loaded and thus trigger inflammation in the small, air-filled cavities of your sinuses (see page 219). They also cause irritation to the eyes and throat. Conventional treatment options mostly include over-the-counter or prescription antihistamines to prevent the onset of allergic reactions, and prescription corticosteroids to reduce inflammation. For more persistent or severe reactions, one may consider immunotherapy – the process, much like homeopathy, of being exposed to small amounts of pollen over a long time period (months to years) to build up a resistance. Including locally produced honey in your diet easily does this. Local is key, as the local bee will have visited every local plant.

Top tip

Cover up when pollen is in the air. Sunglasses, wide-brimmed hat and long sleeves are essential personal protection equipment for sufferers.

Garden treatments

Many plants have low or no pollen – think doubles and sterile hybrids – so you can garden in a low allergy way. There are also plants that alleviate symptoms or prep the body – out of season – for attacks to come. Lemon balm, chamomile and lavender are helpful aromatherapeutic mechanisms to calm allergic reaction. They can also be used throughout the year (not just in seasonal situations) as tisanes to stimulate the body's immunity to allergens. Yarrow, marshmallow, echinacea, eyebright, goldenrod, elderflower and cramp bark all help as infusions or tinctures to alleviate congestion, inflammation and sensitivity. Further antihistaminic constituents are found

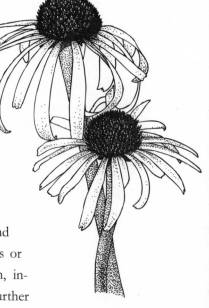

Echinacea

in echinacea, ginkgo, lemon balm and nettle. Witch hazel extract is great for eye treatments.

Kitchen support

Local honey offers good immunology potential – imported honey will have missed the botanical bounty of your region. Histamine is a chemical we naturally produce as a defence mechanism in immune response, as well as being a natural neurotransmitter. In some responses (insect sting, urticaria, allergy, etc.) it does too good a job and the defence inflammation causes as much irritation as the trigger. Antihistamine agents serve to reduce or eliminate that side effect. The best natural antihistamines are contained in the flavonoids that colour our fruits and vegetables, and in the phytochemicals in many herbs and edible plants. Antihistaminic constituents are found in apples/ apple cider vinegar, aronia berries, basil, bell peppers, broccoli, blueberries, cabbage and kale, capers, cranberries, fennel, garlic, ginger, green tea, onions, radishes, raspberries, sweet potatoes, thyme, tomatoes and natural probiotic yoghurt. Bromelain is an anti-inflammatory compound sourced from pineapples (flesh and juice), which also reduces fluid retention and irritation in the nasal membranes and boosts the absorption of other foodstuff and herbal anti-inflammatories. A saline nasal rinse is beneficial too (see page 221).

In The Pink Drink

Four ingredients to boost immunology, address nasal inflammation, increase antihistamine action and energise.

Ingredients

- 1 beetroot or 1 cup beet juice
- 1 pineapple
- 1 tablespoon honey
- 7 marshmallow flowers (or alternately 1 teaspoon any herbal antihistamine from 'Garden treatments')

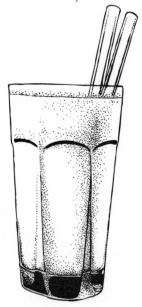

Method

Peel and quarter the beetroot. Peel and dice the pineapple. In a juicer, blender or food processor, add all the ingredients and whizz up a delicious and health-boosting beverage. The juicer will yield juice, the blender a thicker, smoothie-type drink. Chill to serve and enjoy.

HEADACHES

Headaches can vary widely in type and intensity. Medical students learn that there are two sorts of headaches: *primary headaches* – those manifesting without underlying health problems (such as a tension headache), and *secondary headaches* – those with a separate cause or implicated by illness. We could include in the latter a sinus headache and a hangover headache. Within those groups there are subgroups defined by how the pain manifests – cluster, tension, etc. To simplify, and for the purpose of finding the best remedy for the trigger points of each sort of headache, I will explore six categories of headache: tension, cluster, migraine, hormonal, sinusitis and sensitivity. Over-the-counter and garden-grown painkillers will help subdue the pain of all types, but this way we can hit our target much more accurately.

On average, 90 per cent of headaches are due to tension; the other 10 per cent may be hormonal or connected to a cold or condition. But some of us do suffer from migraine or cluster headaches on a regular basis and such recurring headaches deserve more than salicylic acid from meadowsweet or in your foil-packed aspirin. That said, for temporary headaches you can't go wrong with sally (*salix spp*) or feverfew, which has both analgesic and inflammatory properties – unless you're on blood-thinning meds; if so, the garden supplies many solutions and I will explore those in each entry. In the meantime, if you are not sure what is causing your headache, or know with absolute certainty that it is just a standard one, triggered by a late night, hangover, flu side effect, traffic jam or other incident, then rosemary tea helps regulate blood pressure, including intracranial blood pressure, and reduces inflammation and pain sensitivity.

TENSION HEADACHES

Tension headaches fall into two categories: chronic and episodic. If you experience headaches on fifteen or more days per month over several months then you have chronic tension headaches – pain management and stress reduction are the direction you need to take. If you experience them sporadically or less frequently, then they are episodic tension headaches. The tension can be emotional tension or psychological stress, triggering the sensation of an ever-tightening rubber band around the brow and a dull ache inside the skull, or the physical tension exerted by muscle contraction in the neck and head, caused by poor posture or the tenseness stress brings. You may notice that this type often commences at the back of your head and then spreads forward to temples and forehead.

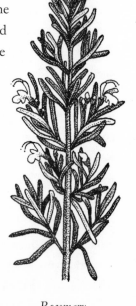

Rosemary

In terms of stress triggers, it is not all about making the mortgage or missing the bus – it can be the stress your system is already under. I know this jumps the primary–secondary barrier, but having conditions such as hypertension or hypoglycaemia can also trigger those rubber-band headaches. The answer is to address the stress and reduce the tension – so a little time out to massage some rosemary or lavender essential oil into the neck and back of the head, or using gentle concentric circles and light massage movements on the temples, will bring the physical and psychological tension down.

Garden treatments

Before we look at the medicinal botany, consider the garden itself. It is a healing tool in its own right, as it encourages a relaxation response. Ignore the ten-storey weeds and just take a little stroll or have a seat. Admire the view but as you do consciously and physically drop your shoulders – I say 'consciously' as this is you psychologically shifting gears. You may have to clunk down a few cogs, as when tense we often raise our shoulders or 'hunch up'. Now with improved posture, breathe deeply. Rest your hands on your belly if you need to, breathe from your diaphragm and fill up your lungs. The surge of fresh oxygen will replenish you and not only help relax your mind and body further, but it will also get your circulatory system to flush toxins out and oxygenated blood in. Whether you practice mindfulness or not, do follow your breath in, and breathe out for a few moments. Clear your thoughts, relax and absorb some positive energy.

As for the herbs, feverfew inhibits the production and release of serotonin and prostaglandins – two significant inflammatory substances that contribute to pain perception and blood-vessel spasm and constriction. Valerian is a muscle relaxant and sedative, which also interrupts and reduces the transmission of pain signals. Passionflower tea and fruit also exert a sedative effect on the central nervous system and relieve both muscle tightening and psychological responses to stress. (See more on stress, page 237.) Corydalis, known as *yan husuo* in traditional Chinese medicine, has been lauded and its analgesic actions compared to those of codeine and morphine. Other natural analgesics include meadowsweet, fennel, St John's wort, wood betony and willow. The fragrance of lavender and chamomile eases tension and is often used by aromatherapists to treat tension headaches.

Willow

Kitchen support

Substance P is the very bland name for a molecule within the body that is far from insipid, as it amplifies pain perception. Phytochemicals in chillies and cayenne pepper (notably capsaicin) deplete it – so a spicy meal may be an effective analgesic. Certain foods have the potential to trigger tension headaches, including chocolate, cheese and dairy, nuts, MSG and fermented foods. You may notice your own particular trigger. If not, you can practise an elimination diet, which generally means eliminating all the potential danger foods, then one by one over several weeks reintroducing them one at a time to see which do trigger headaches – thereafter, delete those items from the grocery list.

Unwind Bath Salts

Lavender is potently adaptogenic, while chamomile is calming – bath delivery is excellent for aroma and skin absorption. The magnesium released from the Epsom salt is soothing to muscle tension and a warm bath is an opportunity in itself to de-stress.

Ingredients

- 2 cups Epsom salt
- 1 cup baking soda
- ½ cup sea salt
- ½ cup lavender flowers (previously sun-dried for several days)
- 2 shakes essential oil of lavender
- 4 shakes essential oil of chamomile

Method

Put all the dry ingredients into a zip-lock or resealable freezer bag, seal and shake well. Add the lavender essential oil, reseal and shake well. Repeat twice more, with two shakes of chamomile oil each time. Spread the contents of the bag onto a sheet of wax paper or baking parchment and allow to air dry for approximately 1 hour – stir about midway. Some aroma will evaporate but it will hold on to a lot too. Store in airtight containers. Use as required (2–3 tablespoons for a bath).

CLUSTER HEADACHES

Cluster headaches are considered primary headaches – they get their name because they are experienced in clusters over a few weeks to a couple of months and then generally disappear for several months to a year. They are cyclical, quite debilitating and painful, often with referred pain around one eye. Over-the-counter painkillers often fail to deaden the intensity of attacks and, while garden or herbal analgesics can take the edge off, the best course of action may be to tackle the mechanisms of manifestation (inflammation, spasm and tension) as a way to pain relief.

Cluster-headache sufferers often have lower than average levels of melatonin. Rectify that by letting day be bright and night be dark. Getting some good daytime exposure (blue wavelength light) promotes a regular circadian rhythm and the appropriate release of melatonin at night. Melatonin production and release is triggered and increased by darkness – invest in blackout curtains and ditch the digital alarm clocks and night lights.

Garden treatments

The garden's anti-inflammatories include birch leaf tea, chamomile, meadowsweet, fennel, feverfew, peppermint, rosemary, slippery elm and black cohosh, while antispasmodics include basil, catnip, cramp bark, hawthorn, juniper berries and spearmint. Poor sleep is a big trigger for cluster headaches – passionflower, valerian, skullcap and Californian poppy will help with that.

Kitchen support

Foods that naturally contain melatonin include bananas, barley and oats, morello cherries, tomatoes, rice, radishes and ginger. Tryptophan helps us make serotonin, which is required to produce and activate melatonin – soy, nuts, sunflower seeds and sesame seeds will boost that component.

Decluster Tea Blend

This tea has anti-inflammatory and antispasmodic constituents.

Ingredients
- Equal quantities of birch leaf, hawthorn leaf and meadowsweet
- Fennel or mint to your personal taste

Method

Stage 1 – how to dry herbs: both birch and hawthorn leaves are best harvested in spring and sun-dried or spread in a thin layer on parchment paper in a pre-heated oven (180°C) with the heat off and the door open. Allow to sit for 20 minutes, turn and sit for a further 20. The other herbs can also be either sun- or oven-dried. Dried herbs can be crumbled and mixed together – if stored in an airtight container they will stay viable for many months.

Stage 2 – to make a tea: add 1 teaspoon of the mix to a tea ball or tea bag and place in a cup of boiling water to infuse for 7–10 minutes.

Restful Night Tea Blend

Poor sleep is a big trigger for cluster headaches; this sedative blend is soothing and analgesic.

Ingredients
- Equal parts by volume of passionflower (both flowers and leaves are suitable – traditionally sun-dried) and Californian poppy (leaves, stems and flowers are all usable – traditionally air-dried in the shade).

Method
Crumble, tear or chop the dried parts to the same size proportionally and place in an airtight container. Shake well. One tablespoon of this blend to 1 cup of boiling water is potent.

MIGRAINE

Migraine is a one-sided throbbing headache caused by constriction and dilation of blood vessels in the brain. The pain is actually caused by the dilation. It also often involves referred eye pain. For a lot of us it's a hereditary condition, but it can develop without a family history. It can be triggered by fluctuations in light levels, noise levels and even temperature. Stress and hormonal fluxes can precipitate it too. There are two types of migraine – common and classical. Nausea and vomiting (see page 204) can attend both. Some people experience such intense migraine that neither herb nor over-the-counter medicines can help. Prescription medications can be discussed with your GP.

Common: persists for a few hours to a few days. Movement and noise seem to intensify the experience.

Classical: can persist for days rather than hours, often preceded by an 'aura' – a visual precursor – blurred vision, flashing lights, a blind spot and sensitivity to light. I find with my own migraines that the signal is olfactory – I smell a sulphurous odour that nobody else can detect.

Garden treatments

Rosemary taken internally regulates blood pressure, including intracranial pressure, and can ease the symptoms of migraine. Feverfew, as the name suggests, can help address fevers, but it is also the standard herb for headaches of all hues – the phytoconstituents in its leaves are analgesic and, especially beneficial for migraines, act to slowly relax blood vessels and ease blood flow. The foliage can be taken in a salad or sandwich, or as a tea or tincture. Meadowsweet is an analgesic and chamomile is calming. Linden tea is sedative and slightly analgesic and has an ethnobotanical history with migraine. The anti-inflammatories and antispasmodics listed under cluster headaches (see page 154) are also remedial for migraine tension in head and neck muscles. Aromatherapeutically, lavender, lemon balm, rosemary and peppermint can be sniffed direct from the garden, utilised as steam baths or, if of the essential sort, used in massage blends. I personally find lavender most effective.

Kitchen support

Foods can trigger migraine in some sufferers, including any food with the amino acid tyrosine/tyramine, e.g. cheese, eggs, bananas, oranges, tomatoes, spinach, soy sauce and – sit down for the next two – wine and chocolate. Tyrosine/tyramine regulates blood pressure, impacts upon constriction and dilation, and signals the brain to release more norepinephrine, which in itself can trigger a headache. Lessen the intake of these foods on a weekly basis and avoid altogether during episodes.

Some foods can diminish migraine patterns – for example migraines are associated with decreased levels of serotonin. To increase the production of serotonin we can avail of the amino acid 5-HTP, which is produced naturally when we eat tryptophan-rich foods such as potato, pumpkin flesh and seeds, sunflower seeds and poultry such as turkey or chicken. Other serotonin boosters include kiwi fruit, bananas, sour cherries, pineapples and plums, tomatoes, turnip, dark green veg and seaweed.

Linden, Lemon Balm and Feverfew Iced Tea or Tincture

When life gives you lemons make lemonade. When life or the garden gives you a headache, reach for the lemon balm, linden and feverfew.

To make an iced tea: simply make as you would a hot tea but on a jug rather than cup scale, using equal parts of the chopped foliage of each plant. Allow to cool for 30 minutes to fully extract the plant phytochemicals. Strain the solids away and then chill the liquid in the fridge. Once chilled, sip throughout the day for the duration of the symptoms.

To make a tincture: fill a jam or mason jar as much as you can (halfway or to the top) with a ratio of equal parts of each herb – chopped – then fill the jar with vodka to immerse the foliage. Lid, label and sit in a sunny place for four weeks. Give it a good shake every few days. Finally strain away the solids and store in a dark glass bottle in a cool, dark place. Tinctures can last indefinitely but I generally review after three years. The dosage is half a teaspoon in some water on the half hour for the duration of the symptoms.

HORMONE HEADACHES (FEMALE SPECIFIC)

Oestrogen actually has some regulatory effects upon brain chemistry and the perception of pain – a drop in levels before menstruation can trigger what are often dubbed 'period migraines'. Hormonal dips and surges around pregnancy, menopause and sometimes related to the contraceptive pill can also trigger headaches. See migraine on page 156, as the treatments for that are also helpful.

Garden treatments

Sage is exceptionally good at calming hormonally triggered headaches – with the knock-on benefit of quelling hot flushes, sweating and irritability. Lavender, as an adaptogenic herb, can balance mood and even out neuroreceptor over-activity – less tension, less headache. Californian poppy and peony have a long history of use for PMS headaches. The gamma-linolenic acid in evening primrose oil and borage oil is very helpful in addressing the diminutions in inhibitory neurotransmitter systems that occur with hormonal fluxes and so head headaches off at the pass. Getting some natural blue wavelength light from daytime outdoor activity or even inactivity – e.g. sitting on a bench – will help reset your circadian rhythms, which have a role in hormone production and release, and will also facilitate a better night's sleep and stronger stress responses next day.

Kitchen support

Sesame seeds have magnesium, a muscle relaxant and relaxer of headaches too, but more importantly they are packed with vitamin E, which supports stability in oestrogen levels. Pumpkin and sunflower seeds are also high in vitamin E – as are many other nuts and seeds. Try more avocados, butternut squash, kiwi, mangos, spinach and broccoli too. Incorporate sage at meal times.

Sage and Shallot Sauce

A delicious delivery of quercetin and pyridoxine – to balance hormonal reactions, raise gamma-amino-butyric acid (good mood chemical) levels and calm irritability and stress.

Ingredients

- ½ cup shallots
- 3 tablespoons chopped, fresh sage
- 1 tablespoon butter
- 1 tablespoon soya oil
- ⅓ glass red wine
- ⅔ cup whipping cream

Method

De-skin and finely chop the shallots. Chop or shred the sage. Melt the butter in a frying pan or skillet, then add the oil and shallots and sauté for 20 seconds, before stirring through the sage. Add the wine and cream and bring to a boil, stirring constantly. Reduce the heat and simmer for 3–5 minutes to allow the sauce to reduce. Serve textured (great with pasta) or hand blend to a smooth consistency.

Bouquet Garni

A culinary staple with medicinal properties. A bundle of equal parts thyme, bay leaves and sage (sometimes also parsley) all tied with string and utilised to make stocks, soups, sauces and casseroles.

SINUS HEADACHE

Sinusitis (see page 219) is an infection or inflammation of the mucous membranes of the nasal cavities, which leads to a build-up of pressure behind the nose (ethmoid sinus), within the head (sphenoid sinus) and around the eyes (frontal sinus) and cheekbone area (maxillary sinus). Prolonged pressure can trigger headaches – often akin to tension headaches. Some argue that it is more of a 'face ache' than a headache – it's all about where that pressure is referring the pain alarm. Sinusitis can manifest because of a cold (see page 64), flu (see page 67) or seasonal allergy such as hay fever (see page 145). Treating the infection will treat the symptoms, so while many of the herbs mentioned here will have varying levels of analgesic qualities, the aim is to hit inflammation and also clear or drain mucus.

Is it really a sinus headache? Sinus headaches and sinus pressure sensations become worse or more throbbing with bending over or lying down, as gravity impacts upon the sinus system. Migraines and tension headaches generally do not.

Garden treatments

A steam inhalation is good for sinus headaches – it clears the build-ups (both mucus and pressure) and is also soothing and anti-inflammatory. Try rosemary, lavender, coriander seeds and eucalyptus. On inhaling eucalyptus, one of its volatile compounds, cineole ($C_{10}H_{18}O$), will also stimulate the immune system. Butterbur is a long-standing remedy for allergies and sinus conditions but an extract is not easy to make at home with complete safety, yet something like feverfew is simple and safe and acts to inhibit the production and release of histamine. Other good antihistamines include nettle, parsley, fennel, evening primrose oil, echinacea and thyme. See also decongestants on pages 60–2.

Kitchen support

Drink fluids. Eat vitamin-C-rich fruits. Spicy meals can help clear sinuses. Ginger and turmeric are useful in dealing with decongestion, pain, inflammation and any attending nausea. Horseradish is powerfully decongestant. Pineapples (juice and flesh) help decrease inflammation in the human body including in the sinuses. Quercetin – available in capsule form in your local health store and naturally available in bright fruits and vegetables – inhibits the production and release of histamine too. A nasal rinse (see page 221) with some table salt can clear out mucus, diminish bacterial infection and remove allergy-triggering particles.

Spicy Nettle and Potato Broth

To clear the head and add antihistamines and analgesics.

Ingredients

- ½ cup nettles
- 1 potato
- 3 cups water
- 1 teaspoon paprika or cayenne pepper
- 1 teaspoon grated or ground ginger
- 1 teaspoon turmeric
- 1 tablespoon chopped chives
- Salt and pepper to taste

Method

Wilt the nettles in a steamer. Peel and dice the potato. Roughly chop the nettles. Cook all the ingredients together until the potatoes are soft. Serve as is, or whizz with a hand blender to a finer soup consistency.

Quick Fix Mustard Footbath

To drain pressure from the head.

Method

Add 1 tablespoon of mustard powder to a basin of warm water. Soak your feet for 15–20 minutes.

SENSITIVITY AND SEASONAL ALLERGY HEADACHES

Sensitivity headaches are those that can be linked to allergies, both environmental (hay fever or too much sun) and food related. Sensitivity headaches can also accompany hangovers, where diminished hydration and toxic build-up in the bloodstream heighten reactions to noise and light, and factor into epilepsy, ADHD and a range of underlying conditions. Sometimes migraines originate as, or are triggered by, increased sensitivity to light or noise. Strain on optic nerves, especially ongoing or repetitive – including screen fatigue – can induce sensitivity headaches, as can food intolerance.

Garden treatments

Antihistamine action from the garden can include nettle, gingko, elderberry, basil, fennel, echinacea, chamomile and butterbur. Butterbur has a long history in Native American ethnobotany – it contains phytochemicals that relieve inflammation and spasms and has applications for a range of conditions. It is quite effective for allergies and sensitivity reactions, but it is not an extract I would attempt to manufacture at home from the garden, as butterbur also contains pyrrolizidine alkaloids (PAs) that can harm the liver over time. The good news is many health stores stock standardised butterbur extracts certified and labelled 'PA-free'.

Kitchen support

Address what you eat, have an allergy test or try omitting a food completely from your diet for a two-week period to detect if it is a trigger. Common triggers include wheat, dairy, chocolate, carbonated drinks, MSG, fermented foods (cheeses, sour cream, etc.), excess sugar and excess salt.

A Cuppa Joe

Coffee – the one with caffeine – can trigger headaches in some, mainly because they have consumed quite a lot. But coffee also works to alleviate two types of headache: migraine to a degree, and seasonal allergy sensitivities to a greater degree. Caffeine is a vasoconstrictor and will reduce the size of blood vessels, thus slowing the pound and throb of a migraine or sensitivity attack. One cup is enough. With seasonal allergies, coffee impedes the release of reactive histamine. It may not be for everyone but it may be for you. Try it and see.

HEARTBURN
(ACID INDIGESTION)

Heartburn is a result of gastric reflux – where the contents of the stomach (digestive enzymes, hydrochloric acid and sometimes food) backflow through the digestive tract causing a burning sensation along the oesophagus. It has nothing to do with your heart – correctly it is acid ingestion – but as it's experienced above the stomach in the chest and breastbone area, we get heart + burn. If frequent it can be symptomatic of GERD (see page 40); if infrequent it can be a reaction to spicy foods, overindulging in food or alcohol, eating on the go while stressed or under pressure, or eating too late to digest before sleep. It is common in pregnancy even without dietary implications. It is implicated in hiatus hernias also.

Garden treatments

Aloe vera juice is soothing to the intestinal tract and neutralises stomach acid, but requires dilution with green tea or water to lessen its laxative properties. Marshmallow root addresses both reflux and digestive disorders as it helps provide a protective layer to the stomach and the oesophagus walls. Meadowsweet tea can help neutralise stomach acids and slow spasms. Many of the digestive herbs not only speed digestion but have antispasmodic actions – try thyme, basil, peppermint, fennel, rosemary and also chamomile, catnip and lemon balm, which help tone the system and exert soothing effects on the stomach too.

Over-the-counter antacids can reduce nutrient absorption, especially of iron, and increase blood pressure. Specific herbal antacids include mint, especially peppermint (more pronounced in its diaphoretic, or perspiration-inducing, action), ginger root, meadowsweet, dandelion and hops. Carminatives (see page 100), apart from helping with digestive distress, are also utilised to assuage oesophageal pressure and relieve heartburn.

Kitchen support

Papaya and liquorice have a long herbal history in treating heartburn and stomach and oesophagus conditions. Potato broth is a traditional reliever, as is milk, but milk long-term can raise gastric juices – OK for the day after curry fest but not if the symptoms are GERD-related. Regular yoghurt may work better. Not all spices are bad – in fact cinnamon and cardamom are antacid. Cabbage water is also traditional – it's alkaline and the glutamine it contains is a calmative, digestively speaking. Magnesium is beneficial and can be sourced in pumpkin and sesame seeds, Brazil, almond and pine nuts, dark leafy veg and also in the rainbow palette of Swiss chard as well as through avocados, bananas and figs. As a quick fix, baking soda will neutralise stomach acid.

ALKALISING FOODS

Vegetables: artichokes, beetroot, broccoli, Brussels sprouts, carrots, cauliflower, celery, courgette, cucumber, green beans, kale, lettuce, radishes, peas, peppers, potatoes, spinach, squash, turnip and watercress

Fruits: apples, avocados, bananas, berries, grapes, melon, peaches, pears and watermelon

Protein: almonds and other nuts, pumpkin seeds, sunflower seeds, tofu and soya products

---

Bicarb, Epsom and Peppermint Julep (minus the alcohol)

OK, it's not technically a julep – there is no bourbon – but it is a 'smash' (a type of cocktail that juleps originated from). Smashes often involve the muddling (crushing and agitating to release volatile oils and flavours) of a herb at the bottom of the serving glass. We are doing the same but for its healing ingredients as well flavour.

Method
Put 1 teaspoon each of bicarbonate of soda, Epsom salt and peppermint into a tall glass, muddle, then add two-thirds of a glass of water and stir well.

Minty Marshmallow and Meadowsweet Antacid

All ingredients are naturally alkaline or directly antacid in action.

Method

Overnight in the fridge, cold infuse half a cup of meadowsweet tops in a cup of soya milk. Strain away the solids and blitz in a blender with 2 mint leaves and one-third of a cup of marshmallow flowers. Keeps in the fridge for three to four days. Sip or drink as required. Good after a meal.

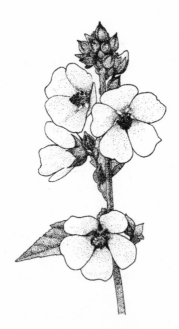

Marshmallow flower

HICCUPS

A hiccup is an audible effect of the vocal chords caused by an involuntary contraction of the diaphragm that is out of sync with the capacity of your windpipe to respond. The contraction causes an inhalation, but the glottis blocks the breath. That contraction and its audible side effect are easily triggered by eating too much, too fast, consuming carbonated beverages or overindulgence in alcohol. Some hiccups are triggered by sudden changes in temperature and some by excitement or stress. Hiccups resolve naturally shortly after commencement, but if you are a frequent hiccuper then the following might help to relieve them.

Garden treatments

Holding your breath indoors or outdoors builds up carbon dioxide in the bloodstream and halts hiccups by inhibiting spasms. It's not a *Guinness Book of Records* job – don't pass out – just take a deep breath, hold it longer than normal, exhale, hold again a little while, then breathe normally. Repeat a few cycles and the hiccups should dissipate. Or you can pull your knee up to your chest to exercise the spasming diaphragm. The scare trick only works if it distracts the brain or incites the vagus nerve, which is implicated in hiccups, but eating sweet foods and, for some, smelling strong smells, can also stimulate the vagus. So munch a strawberry and smell the roses.

Kitchen support

Drinking a glass of water can hack the signals of the vagus nerve, which runs from the brain to the stomach, and shut down hiccup messages. You don't have to drink upside down, which is the old husbands' tale (why should wives get all the blame!). Sampling something sweet – a spoonful of honey or a finger lick of jam – does the same trick.

Nectar Tea

A simple sweet treat to usurp the hiccup.

Method

Simply add 1 tablespoon of honey and some edible petals of your choice to a cup of boiling water. Allow to infuse over several minutes until cool enough to sip – use the fridge to speed up the process.

HOT FLUSHES

A sudden sensation of warmth or heat in the face and neck, or perception of a whole body temperature rise, is known as a hot flush – it is a very common symptom of the menopause and occasionally accompanies pregnancy. Sometimes hot sensations are accompanied by dizziness or nausea (see page 204). In general hot flushes can last from a couple of minutes to half an hour, a couple of times a week to several times a day. Duration and intensity varies from person to person. While the symptoms are similar, the treatment regimens differ between menopausal and pregnancy-related flushes.

MENOPAUSAL HOT FLUSHES

Drops in oestrogen levels seem to impede the correct functioning of the hypothalamus (the brain's thermostat), which senses body temperature, and so blood is flushed into the face and neck heightening heat perception. Also decreasing levels of oestrogen alter the body's response to stress and cause more norepinephrine and epinephrine to be released into the bloodstream, which increases blood flow and can raise temperature in sudden surges that may also be experienced as hot flushes.

Garden treatments

Sage tea is perfect for menopausal flush and has been employed for thousands of years to quell both hot flushes and night sweats. Likewise parsley can regulate hormones. Both contain oestrogen-like compounds that attach to oestrogen receptors in the body and give the impression of higher levels, which tricks the hypothalamus into functioning effectively. Other phytoestrogen herbs include angelica/dong quai, black cohosh, evening primrose, liquorice root, ginseng and red clover. Black cohosh tea is a traditional remedy for night sweats (see page 115). Chamomile promotes good sleep and helps to de-stress in waking hours, while motherwort is often utilised to treat palpitations that accompany hot flushes. Gamma linolenic acid (GLA) – sourced from evening primrose oil, blackcurrant seed oil, borage oil and also from health stores (including hemp seed oil) – is the precursor for prostaglandin PGE1, which helps regulate hormonal balance and can address hot flushes and other menopausal reactions.

Kitchen support

Hydration is a great starting point, so drink plenty of water and/or herbal teas. Eat more phytoestrogen-rich foods such as alfalfa, barley, dried beans, lentils, flaxseed, sesame seeds, wheatgerm, rice bran, apples, carrots, pomegranates, berries, oats and walnuts. One of the best choices is soybean, which contains two significantly oestrogenic compounds, genistein and daidzein; these can also help slow osteoporosis. Foods with magnesium and calcium help by alkalising the system and cutting out acidic foods can lessen attacks too. Foods best avoided to decrease frequency or intensity of hot flushes include alcohol, caffeine, sugar and spicy food. It is worth noting that prostaglandin synthesis requires not just GLA but also zinc and magnesium, vitamin C, vitamin B6 and niacin – all easily sourced from foods.

Perfect Sage Tea

There is a trick to making the perfect sage tea: infuse the herb in water that has been boiled but rested for a minute, as boiling water can damage some of the phytochemical and volatile oils but hot water will extract them intact. When it comes to ratios, fresh and dry vary – so if fresh use 2 tablespoons to each cup; if dried 1 tablespoon will do. Fresh or dried, it is good idea to cover with a saucer when infusing to retain more of the volatile oils and allow to steep for 10 minutes. Honey and/or lemon can be added to flavour. Sage tea can also be iced.

PREGNANCY HOT FLUSHES

Hormonal fluxes during pregnancy can cause the sensation of a heat flush to face and neck. Pregnancy flushes are experienced by one in ten pregnant women and can become more consistent in the second and third trimesters and remain a while after delivery – especially if breastfeeding. Any oestrogen-level drop disrupts the hypothalamus. Most flushes last two to three minutes, but some can last up to half an hour. They are self-resolving, but a fan or a cool drink does no harm. If they are becoming problematic (overly frequent), then there are some safe options to explore and some unsafe ones to avoid.

Garden treatments

Both parsley and sage tea are synonymous with quelling hot flushes but, while perfectly acceptable to address menopausal flush, when it comes to pregnancy it's a different matter. Parsley is an emmenagogue and can trigger uterine contractions, while sage tea contains thujone, a molecule that can raise blood pressure – so **AVOID BOTH**. Likewise herbal iced teas are cooling, but many herbs have the potential to stimulate the uterus, so avoid lime blossom, rose hip, catnip, chamomile, comfrey, hibiscus, horehound, liquorice root, mugwort, raspberry leaf, rosemary, nettle and yarrow. Instead think green tea.

Mindfulness techniques and exercises, in the garden or anywhere, will generate more positive actions in the amygdala, the portion of the brain in charge of emotional response and proportional adrenaline release, which also affects temperature perception. Smell a nice herb, follow your breath, visualise your lawn as a tropical beach with the warm waves ebbing and flowing against your toes.

Kitchen support

Drink plenty of water to keep hydrated or rehydrate if flushes are encouraging sweating. Think isotonic beverages or electrolyte-rich coconut water if the latter. Phytoestrogens such as soy and seeds can alleviate symptoms. Calcium-rich and magnesium-rich foods support stable temperatures and stress responses too.

A Cup of Green Tea

A cup of green tea is good to go and even better outdoors where the garden can have a relaxation response on the mind–body–spirit. Best of all it can affect your amygdala too. The natural compound L-theanine found in green tea promotes relaxing alpha waves in the brain and alters brain chemistry by raising both dopamine levels and gamma-amino-butyric acid production – all of which supports increased serotonin (happy hormone) levels and a sense of well-being.

Method
Make as normal – no milk or sugar. Delicious chilled with lemon slices.

INSOMNIA

Insomnia is the inability to sleep or the experience of poor quality and quantity of sleep. It can be considered *acute* or *chronic*. *Acute* or short-term insomnia generally lasts a single night or a short cluster of a few nights over a week or more. *Chronic* is the complication extending into repeated bouts over several weeks and, in the extreme, over several months.

Acute insomnia can be a simple case of environmental factors such as noise (traffic, rattling wind, a party next door), light (brightness keeps the mind alert) or temperature (hot or cold can impact on the body's ability to rest). It can be occasioned by illness or physical discomfort and even conventional treatments for those conditions (some medications can interrupt normal sleep patterns). It can also be occasioned by emotional discomfort (stress, office politics and unrequited love, alas, can all play on the mind at night) and similarly medications to address anxiety and depression can have sleep-altering side effects. Shift work, jet lag and so on can also trigger short-term insomnia.

Chronic or prolonged insomnia most often pertains to chronic stress, depression or anxiety, or to an underlying ailment causing night-time bodily discomfort or mental anguish.

Whichever you suffer from, insomnia can be a vicious circle in that anxiety and fear of not sleeping generates more anxiety and adrenaline to psychologically and chemically undermine the sleep potential. Sleep is essential for brain function and cellular regeneration, so loss of it impacts directly upon health and daily function. Insomnia upsets the natural balance, cognitive performance and our hormonal rhythms but it, and its ancillary symptoms of fatigue (see page 123), irritability and stress (see page 237), can be treated and reversed.

Garden treatments

Both chamomile and lavender are the go-to herbs for rest and sleep. Clip a little of either one and smell it, put some in the bath or sip a tisane of it – both steady the nerves, counter stress and even out the excesses of caffeine and biochemicals that keep you from peaceful rest. Cowslip petal tea is sedative and soothing to the mind. Valerian root harvested for tea or tincture is sedative and hypnotic (the latter meaning sleep-inducing rather than making you walk like a duck or believe you are naked) and it also helps alleviate spontaneous fidgeting and muscle spasms that can be a part of a restless night. Passionflower is both sedative and antispasmodic, and suitable in tea or tincture form. Other sedative herbal teas include those made from linden flowers, Californian poppy and hops; mood-enhancing and rest-inducing herbs include lavender, lemon balm, catmint and skullcap. All those mentioned are also considered to be anxiolytic (anti-anxiety) herbs.

Kitchen support

Eating at night is not good for the waistline, but if your insomnia is short term then a midnight feast might just tip the scales in your favour. Lettuce is considered a natural night-time sedative, but there are benefits in tryptophan-rich foods such as milk, cheese, bananas and other sources of protein. Tryptophan is a neurotransmitter in human physiology that regulates sleep and slightly sedates you after ingestion. A cup of tea (green or black) contains L-theanine, a neurologically active amino acid that stimulates the production of alpha brain waves, thus inducing a relaxing effect. It won't make you drowsy or fall asleep, but its anxiolytic potential is good to support you through the day and set you up for a good night's sleep.

TIPS TO TRIGGER SLEEP

1. Avoid naps – keep the tiredness for night-time.
2. Avoid stimulants after 4 p.m. – caffeine, nicotine, etc. can keep you alert and awake.
3. Go dark – bright light (artificial or daylight) inhibits the release of melatonin, the sleep hormone.
4. Get cool – cooler temperatures put the body into rest mode.

A Lavender Pillow

Aromatherapy while you sleep.

1. Getting the lavender: harvest when in bloom and early in the morning. Cut into the green, not the woody, part of the plant. Take enough of the stem to leave leaves behind but with enough length to easily hang the stalks. You can of course dry individual stalks, spaced out on drying racks, but the traditional method of drying in bundles is not only viable but aesthetically pleasing when hung about the house. If you dry in your bedroom then the night-time therapy has already begun. Tie bundles at their base with string or elastic bands and hang upside down in a darkish, dry environment (drying in airing cupboards or inside perforated paper bags helps retain more volatile oils). At room temperature, the bundles will take about four weeks to dry. Thereafter you can run the stalks through your fingers to dislodge the lavender grains (the dried individual flowers). Store in airtight containers or add directly to pre-made sachets.

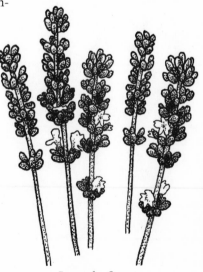

Lavender flowers

2. Making the pillow: we are making a sachet that can be slipped between your pillow and its pillowcase. Take a fabric handkerchief or similar-sized muslin square and fold it in half. Sew a closing seam along the top and one other side to make a pouch. Fill the pouch with lavender grains. Once fully packed (you can add cotton wool to pad if required), sew up the opening. That's it! Pop it into your pillowcase and look forward to a restful night's sleep.

MENSTRUAL CRAMPS (DYSMENORRHEA)

Dysmenorrhea is the medical definition for period pain – cramping pain below the abdomen (but also often extending into the back and other areas). While the intensity and duration of period pain varies from woman to woman, and even from cycle to cycle, there are two types of period pain/menstrual cramp.

Primary dysmenorrhea is the most common type – described as sensitivity to prostaglandins, the role of which in the menstrual cycle is to trigger contractions that facilitate the removal of the lining of the womb: a normal period. The type of prostaglandin that is the problem – F2 alpha – also halts progesterone production. In some women periods can be accompanied by elevated prostaglandin (much more than required) and thus the womb contracts too hard, interfering with both oxygen and blood supply and so generating a pain experience. Primary dysmenorrhea most often occurs in teenagers and women in their twenties. Ancillary symptoms include headache (see page 149), backache (see page 48), fatigue (see page 123), nausea and vomiting (see page 204), constipation (see page 75) or diarrhoea (see page 95) and bloating (see page 102).

Secondary dysmenorrhea is most likely to affect women in their thirties and forties and is a cramp-like experience generated not by hormonal fluxes but by an underlying condition in the womb or pelvis – endometriosis, fibroids, infection or inflammatory disease. Pain may extend into hips, thighs and lower back. Medical intervention for underlying ailments is advised but garden-harvested and kitchen-prepared anti-inflammatories (see page 208), infection busters (see page 70) and painkillers (see page 36) will address symptoms.

Garden treatments

Fennel has a long history of use to reduce hormone fluctuation but best of all it is a powerful antispasmodic. Valerian is a muscle relaxant that also interrupts and reduces the transmission of pain signals. Guelder rose, aka cramp bark, is an antispasmodic and relaxant. Black haw is an antidote to spasm and cramping while black cohosh, beyond its great anti-inflammatory and antispasmodic action, is ideal for pain that radiates to the lower back and pain referred to hips and thighs. Chamomile tea and aroma is anti-inflammatory and antispasmodic. The fragrance of lavender is a powerful mood balancer, while lilac aroma is considered a tranquilliser. Serenity supports pain-experience control – mindfulness exercises rewire the brain for better control too.

Prostaglandin F2 alpha is a known inflammatory, so borage and evening primrose oil not only remedy inflammation via their omega-6 fatty acid but also have been used for centuries to tone the uterus, harmonise energy levels and balance mood and hormones. One cannot overlook the benefits of GLA to the reproductive system in general. As a long-term support, regular utilisation of red raspberry leaf tea can tone the uterus and diminish or prevent menstrual cramps.

Kitchen support

Isotonic drinks can help but one should watch out for more than sodium loss – loss of potassium, magnesium and calcium will also cause an ionic imbalance impacting on normal contraction and expansion of the muscles and intensifying the sensation of cramp and pain. Milk is full of calcium which helps regulate muscle tone and thus assists the relief of cramping – as do almonds, beans and dark green leafy vegetables. Apple cider vinegar is also rich in cramp-easing nutrients and calcium and potassium. Coconut water contains all the electrolytes needed to ease cramp.

Avoid sugary, refined and highly glycaemic foods – all are known to increase prostaglandin F2 alpha levels. Think instead of antioxidants from blueberries, cherries and even sweet tomatoes. One should not underestimate the impact of food upon hormones – a low-fat, high-fibre diet will significantly reduce oestrogen levels and thus reduce cramping. Fibre in particular is useful – where oestrogen is normally extracted from the bloodstream by the liver, a little extra fibre will 'soak up' excesses of oestrogen and remove it as part of normal 'waste disposal'.

Cramp Bark Tea

Cramp bark is a uterine sedative and muscle relaxant that also exhibits astringent and disinfecting properties. The dried bark is available in many health stores or you can harvest and dry it during autumn or spring.

Method

The tradition is to harvest at least two-year-old stems, peel the bark off and dry the strips in an oven at a low heat over a few hours. The tea ratio is generally 1 teaspoon to 1 cup of hot water for a 7–10 minute infusion. Strain away solids before sipping.

MORNING SICKNESS AND HYPEREMESIS GRAVIDARUM

Not all pregnant women will experience the nausea and vomiting known as morning sickness, which occurs most often between the sixth and the twelfth weeks of pregnancy. But it is perfectly normal and related to the presence of the hormone human chorionic gonadotropin (hCG) which supports your growing foetus until the placenta takes over and hCG levels drop and your nausea with it. Those that do suffer will experience it with differing frequencies and intensity. 'Morning sickness' is a bit of a misnomer, as pregnancy-related nausea can occur at any time of the day. Of those who do experience it, it is estimated that 1 in 300 can experience a strong reaction known as hyperemesis gravidarum, which is also a hormone-complicated condition manifesting with severe and regular vomiting that can continue even after the twelfth week. Both sorts cause dehydration, malnutrition (to self and foetus) and weight and energy loss. It is important to get medical supervision with this one.

Garden treatments

Lemon balm and peppermint as tea have settling properties, but some find their aromas too strong during early pregnancy. Fennel tea is antispasmodic and digestive. The chlorophyll and phytonutrients in alfalfa, kelp, spirulina and wheatgrass shots are restorative and antiemetic.

The fresh air of the garden is calming and can settle upsets. The vitamin D of sunshine and the alpha waves of daylight can balance hormones and give a sense of well-being. The green lawn and foliage can lower blood pressure and create a relaxation response. Connecting with nature is a powerful healer – time out is restorative to mind–body–spirit and deeply supportive to a healthy pregnancy.

Kitchen support

Avoid foods and aromas that make you feel nauseated but don't skip meals. Low blood sugar aggravates both morning sickness and hyperemesis gravidarum. B-vitamin-rich foods restrict and alleviate nausea and vomiting – that's a little more wholegrain, brown rice, brewer's yeast, banana and avocado. Ginger is normally antiemetic but its effectiveness in pregnancy-related nausea and sickness is not always assured. Some women who may have had success with ginger in non-pregnancy nausea find that during pregnancy it can trigger heartburn. Others sing its virtues. That's the thing with pregnancy – different strokes.

One thing important for all is maintaining good hydration, as it is important to lessen the experience of nausea and to replenish moisture after vomiting. Sipping iced water or barley water (see page 69) throughout the day is a great option. Coconut water is refreshing and rehydrating, and is great in a smoothie too, as it contains the five electrolytes that your body needs: potassium, sodium, magnesium, phosphorous and calcium. Green tea not only eases morning sickness and calms an upset stomach – all those antioxidants are beneficial for de-stressing and maintaining long-term health. Add a little lemon or honey, as they too have antiemetic value. Sweetness in general is antiemetic, so honey is ideal – even just a lick of the spoon will do the trick. Honey is not dangerous to your unborn child even though it is not recommended as a food source for infants under a year old because unpasteurised and natural honeys may potentially contain spores of harmful bacteria normally destroyed in the adult acidic digestive tract but not in the lesser acidity of a baby's digestive tract.

Simply Banana Gelato

This is a brilliant one-ingredient, simple, delicious gelato-style treat. The pectin and cellular structures of bananas make this a creamy delight.

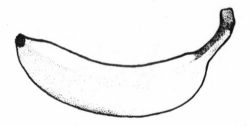

Ingredients
- A very ripe banana or two (that's plenty of freckles).

Method
Peel the banana(s) and slice into circles or chunks to freeze overnight.

Remove the frozen banana from freezer and pop into a food processor or sturdy blender and blitz until it goes a bit gooey. Scrape down the sides of the food processor or blender. Re-blitz a little more, passing through a lumpy porridge stage into full-on smooth, thick custard consistency.

Scoop the blended banana into an airtight container and freeze for an hour or until solid. This keeps in the freezer for weeks – but is eaten in minutes!

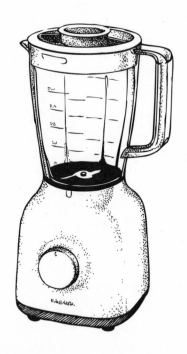

MOUTH ULCERS
(APHTHOUS ULCER)
AND CANKER SORES
(APHTHOUS STOMATITIS)

Mouth ulcers and canker sores are somewhat identical. Stress or tissue injury is thought to be implicated in the development of mouth ulcers – whatever their true type is. In some cases, ulcers are caused by an underlying health condition (especially connected to a weakened immune system or gastrointestinal tract disease). Occasionally the trigger is a nutritional deficiency. Certain foods (mainly acidic fruits) can exacerbate or trigger a flare-up. They are triggered too by hormonal fluctuations or menstrual cycles. Mouth ulcers and canker sores can re-emerge four or more times a year and are not considered contagious (but the virus or bacterial infections start somewhere).

Mouth ulcers: there are several types of mouth ulcers. *Minor ulcers*, the most common type, are generally 2–8mm in diameter, non-scarring and often self-resolving within ten to fourteen days. *Major ulcers* are generally 1cm or more in diameter and usually deeper, with a raised or irregular border. They can leave scarring marks and take many weeks to resolve. *Herpetiform ulcers* are clusters of anywhere from five to a hundred fused pinhead-sized sores. They are painful and often scarring, but rarer than the other types.

Canker sores is a universal term for a type of small painful ulcer of the mouth – defined by being rather craterlike or indented and off-white to yellow with red rims. Canker sores mainly develop on the insides of the cheeks, the gums and inner lips, but can compromise the tongue, oesophagus and gastrointestinal tract.

Garden treatments

Decoctions of lovage root as gargles and rinses have a long history in herbal treatments for mouth sores. There is actually a plant known as canker root (aka goldthread) and a poultice of its raw root or a tisane as a rinse was common in Native American ethnobotany. Alternatively goldenseal was utilised to reduce inflammation of mucous membranes and impart antibacterial action. Barberry and Oregon grape have similar constituents. Aloe vera sap supplies anti-inflammatory salicylates to the mouth and wound site, which also relieve pain. Many herbal teas can fight sores with disinfecting phytochemicals but those highest in tannins can tighten and shrink the craters – try bearberry, eucalyptus, St John's wort, sage, raspberry leaf, rose, mint/peppermint and liquorice. Tannins are wound cleaners. The term tannin comes from the High German tanna, denoting oak or fir trees, so you can make a rinse from some oak or pine bark. I recommend antimicrobials and antiseptics to keep the mouth clean and tackle any underlying infection – try eucalyptus leaves, fennel, lavender, mint, thyme and uva ursi – and immunostimulants such as astragalus root, echinacea, elderberry, meadowsweet and thyme will get to the root of the complaint.

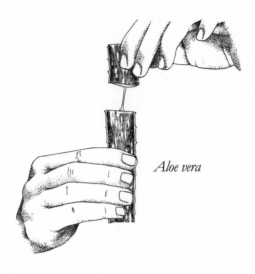

Aloe vera

Kitchen support

Black tea is high in tannins. Garlic is antiviral and antibacterial. As mouth ulcers and mouth sores can pertain to a deficiency of vitamin B12, folic acid, iron or zinc, a well-balanced diet and an increase in whole grains, nuts and cereals can act as supplements. Fruits and foods rich in vitamin C and bioflavonoids will enhance the body's own natural healing mechanisms, but citrus fruits and acidic food can exacerbate the condition. Coconut oil has analgesic, anti-inflammatory and antimicrobial properties (it's also a good base for a few drops of pain-suppressing eugenol found in clove oil and crushed cloves). Honey is antimicrobial and remedial to canker sores and mouth ulcers, and it can be a base for antimicrobials and pain- or inflammation-suppressing items from the spice rack – turmeric, garlic, cinnamon and clove.

Antiseptic Pulling Oil

Coconut oil at room temperature can be swished around the mouth to deliver analgesic lauric acid and also to diminish bacteria and target infections. Infusing it with herbs increases its potency.

Method

In a saucepan of simmering water heat a jam jar half-filled with coconut oil until it melts and warms. Add 1 teaspoon of ground cloves, 1 tablespoon of dried sage and 1 tablespoon of dried and powdered mahonia root. Keep on the heat for 20 minutes. Stir well. Allow to cool and reset. Use a spoonful – it will melt in the mouth – three times daily to swish around the mouth and pull between teeth by sucking it in and out. Spit out after 2–3 minutes of swishing. If you don't like the oily mouth feel, you can brush your teeth as normal afterwards.

MUSCLE ACHES

Muscle aches can have a variety of triggers but mainly cramp, sprain or strains are the culprits.

CRAMP

This is an involuntarily contraction that does not rest for a few moments and can be experienced as a taut soreness or throb of pain, often occasioned by insufficient blood supply to the muscle, dehydration, exertion causing strain or, on occasion, a metabolic or mineral deficiency.

Garden treatments

Black cohosh and cramp bark are two potent antispasmodics employed by most herbalists for repeated cramping, but other possibilities include evening primrose oil, motherwort, nettle and valerian – all of which are antispasmodic with some nervine qualities too. Antispasmodics stop or ease spasm reflex, while nervines soothe the nerves and, by reaction, the muscles involved in the spasm. Common garden nervines include St John's wort, skullcap, valerian and vervain. Gingko and ginger boost circulation. Horse chestnut has value in internal and external applications – tincture for internal, pastes for external.

Eating garden fruits (strawberries, raspberries, aronia, blueberries, apples, etc.) is great for rehydrating the system; purple fruits and veg boost stamina and help muscle recovery, if it's over-exertion that has led to cramping. A few stretches in the garden can resolve cramping in limbs, and partaking of the sedative or soothing fragrance of lilac, lavender, honeysuckle or roses can distract the brain from spasm signals.

Kitchen support

Oats are a great nervine; ginger and garlic work well to tone the circulatory system. Coconut water is a brilliant natural isotonic drink packed with all of the electrolytes needed to revive a dehydrated muscle and soothe post-cramp tissue. When it comes to minerals and muscle spasms, the key ones are sodium, potassium, magnesium and calcium – any deficiency of these can disrupt the balance of ions within the muscle tissues that regulate normal contraction and efficient expansion. We can sweat these out during strenuous activity or just hot-day gardening chores.

We think of drinking to replenish electrolytes but we can eat them too. Cheese and pickles are often high in sodium, so a ploughman's for lunch could set you right – or try a salad or tofu with some sodium-rich soy sauce or add a pinch of table salt to a glass of juice. Fruits and vegetables rich in potassium include avocado, bananas, broccoli, cauliflower, carrots, cucumber, tomatoes, spinach, strawberries and oranges. Magnesium is found in dairy products and also in wholegrain cereal, barley and oats, in black beans, broccoli, soybeans and tofu. Calcium is also found in dairy products and in avocados, carrots, tomatoes, garlic, onions, bananas, grapes, pineapples and leafy green vegetables.

Beetroot and Orange Boost Juice

The vitamin C from oranges is remedial to cramp, while the phytochemicals in beetroot improve muscle recovery. Both boost stamina.

Method
Simply mix equal parts by volume of beetroot juice and orange juice. Drink chilled.

Cool Solution Muscle Rub

Menthol and camphor act as prime relief agents in most over-the-counter cramp treatments. Menthol is a natural constituent of any plant in the mint family and camphor is a natural constituent of coriander, lavender, rosemary, hyssop, oregano and sage.

Ingredients
- 3 tablespoons chopped mint
- 1 tablespoon coriander seeds
- 2 tablespoons chopped hyssop (or other camphor herb)
- 3 tablespoons vodka
- 100ml witch hazel extract

Method
Add all the ingredients to a blender and blitz. Decant to a dark bottle and store in a dark cupboard for three days. You can strain the solids or keep them infusing. Use as required.

STRAIN VERSUS SPRAIN

Muscle strain is not as severe as muscle sprain – it is not about torn or stretched ligaments but the dull ache of an overworked muscle. It is one of the most common gardening complaints and sports injuries. It can manifest as a stiffness and progress to a pain or heaviness in the affected limb or region of the muscle. Rubbing the area flushes blood to the site and speeds the healing process. You may see footballers walking off a light cramp for the same reason. A bit of PRICE (protection, rest, ice, compression and elevation) is helpful in halting further injury. When it comes to the ice part, 15–20 minutes every hour while awake will both numb pain and reduce inflammation. The compression is simply a gently applied elastic bandage which, when combined with elevation, decreases swelling and forces you to rest. We can steal a trick from sports medicine and learn to employ ice packs early while maintaining the strained muscle in a stretched position. Some aches go with the rub, others resolve before you have fetched the ice, but if a strain lingers the following treatments will help.

Garden treatments
A cup of linden flower tea has a slight sedative and thus mildly analgesic effect and it improves blood supply to sore muscles. Gingko also gets the blood moving. Flushing the area with blood will naturally flush away the agents of ache – lactic acid, toxins, haematomas, etc. Meadowsweet tea is a natural aspirin (and also thins the blood), while yarrow and rosemary in topical rubs and

oral application have an affinity with strain recovery. Any garden mint blitzed or mashed up in a little coconut oil (which also decreases pain perception) will provide cooling stimulation to aches when topically applied.

Kitchen support

The capsicum in cayenne pepper and chillies deadens the perception of pain – avail of it by adding either spice to a massage blend to add therapeutic heat to the area or it can be used to spice up your evening meals for a few days. Other helpful spices include pain-relieving turmeric, ginger, cinnamon and cloves.

Sore Muscle Salve

A stimulating and remedying salve for sore muscles, with warming herbs and analgesic and antispasmodic action.

Ingredients

- 10 leaves garden mint
- 20 leaves catmint
- 1 sprig rosemary
- ¼ cup grated ginger
- 1 tablespoon cayenne pepper or 1 teaspoon mustard powder
- 10 cloves
- 1½ cups olive oil or alternative vegetable or nut carrier oil
- 20g unadulterated beeswax

Method

Wash and kitchen-towel dry your harvested herbs, then tear, crush or chop to help release their active principles. Place the herbal parts, ginger and spices into a mason jar and completely cover with the carrier oil. Then put on the lid or seal the opening with cellophane or kitchen parchment. Bring a pan of water to the boil, then turn off the heat. Stand the mason jar in the hot water and let sit to commence infusing. After 30 minutes return the pan to the heat and simmer the infusion receptacle for a further two hours, adding water to the pan as evaporation occurs. Then turn off the heat and allow the receptacle to continue infusing for a further 30 minutes. Decant the oil into a second jar, straining the herb parts away. Chip, shave or grate the beeswax into the hot, infused oil and stir until it dissolves fully and is absorbed (add gentle heat via the bain-marie if needed). Decant the mixed liquid to your storage container and let cool and solidify before lidding and storing for use. This will last for a year if stored in a cool location.

Muscle sprain/pulled muscle/ligament injury is often referred to as a pulled muscle, but it is in fact a ligament injury. Sprains are painful (and debilitating), while strains are closer to an ache (and wear off). Ligaments are the tough straps – quite similar to elastic bands in action – that connect bone to bone and secure joints in place. A sprain results from the tearing of ligament fibres – sometimes partially and sometimes fully. The more intense the pain and the larger the swelling, the more likely it is to be a complete tear, which may necessitate surgery. Including the knee and ankle, where gardeners are prone to develop problems, we have ligaments at every joint.

The best response is to follow the PRICE protocol as mentioned above – protection, rest, ice, compression and elevation. In this instance, with the 'rest' portion being at least forty-eight hours, if no improvements are noted on day three of the injury then visit your GP for evaluation. If the joint feels unstable or numb, then medical assistance should be sought the same day as the injury. PRICE is often complemented by heat packs or sprain plasters on day two and three, but ice or cold packs will take the inflammation down in the first two days.

Garden treatments

A refreshing herbal tea fresh from the garden with plants selected to improve blood flow to damaged structures is the ticket. Blood flow will resolve inflammation quicker by completing healing processes faster. Make a blend of any three of the following: linden flowers, gingko foliage, hawthorn foliage, prickly ash bark and yarrow flowers – all excellent for encouraging peripheral circulation.

Kitchen support

With strong inflammation the body's adrenal glands release the natural anti-inflammatory defence chemical cortisone. Turmeric improves the uptake and absorption of cortisone at sites of stress – include it in a topical compress. You can add it to food too.

Sprained Muscle Plaster

Both horsetail (*Equisetum arvense*) and comfrey have been a part of herbal tissue-repair remedies for centuries – their successful medicinal action is because of the silica content and other phytochemicals that build connective tissues. Both have been taken internally up until recent times but this remedy is for topical application.

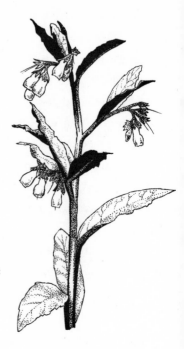

Comfrey

Ingredients

- ½ cup *Equisetum arvense* foliage and stems or 30 drops mother tincture
- ½ cup chopped comfrey foliage and stems or 30 drops mother tincture
- ½ cup chopped birch, salix or ash foliage or 2 crushed aspirin tablets
- ½ cup vinegar
- 3 tablespoons grated ginger
- 3 tablespoons mustard powder
- 1 tablespoon ground turmeric
- Cornflour to thicken or water to loosen

Method

Add all the ingredients, excluding the cornflour or water, to a saucepan and bring to the boil. Put a lid on and rest off the heat for 20 minutes. Whisk with a hand blender. Finally, thicken or loosen by adding cornflour or water if needs be. Once at a comfortable temperature, apply to the sprain – utilise a cling-film bandage to keep it in place if required and leave for 30 minutes before rinsing clean. Repeat applications over a two- to three-day period – if it does not improve, the tear may be in need of medical intervention.

NAUSEA AND VOMITING

Nausea and vomiting are not diseases or ailments; rather they are the symptoms of many conditions from viral infections to stress, from food poisoning to motion sickness, from infection to that 'one for the road' mistake. Nausea is the sick sensation – the feeling you want to vomit. Vomiting is actually getting sick, throwing up, and by its nature it can cause dehydration, making you feel worse and recover more slowly. Nausea is the early warning system that everything is not quite right, while vomiting is the body's attempt to remove harmful agents from the body. One doesn't always lead to the other, but many treatments actually alleviate both symptoms, so we can treat them here as the same. See morning sickness (see page 187) for pregnancy-safe herbs. If you are aware of the contributing factor then look up its entry to treat that cause too – for example, for food poisoning see page 233, for migraine see page 156 and for flu see page 67.

Garden treatments

The garden, with all its fresh air and sunlight, can centre you and bring a sense of well-being as well as control. Breathing deeply can control sensations of nausea and smelling aromatic plants can shift the brain to other perceptions. Of course you can use antiemetic herbs such as fennel, mint and meadowsweet to reduce the feeling of nausea and halt or prevent vomiting. Dandelion, milk thistle, catmint and lemon balm also are traditional remedies for nausea and vomiting – as tea or tinctures. The aromatherapy and tea or tincture of chamomile, lavender and peppermint all settle the stomach, assuage nausea and help recovery post-vomiting. Antispasmodics can also help with the gag reflex and stomach-muscle spasms associated with nausea and vomiting – try black cohosh, evening primrose oil, motherwort, thyme, red clover or valerian.

SEEK IMMEDIATE MEDICAL CARE

If there is blood in the vomit (not always bright red fluid – blood can appear like coffee grounds).

For a head injury, severe headache, stiff neck or crippling abdominal pain.

If there is rapid breathing or accelerated pulse.

If you suspect you have ingested something poisonous.

Kitchen support

Ginger, cloves, lemongrass and dill are culinary antiemetics. Blueberry and other fruits may prevent symptoms of nausea and vomiting due to their phytochemical content and also their sweetness. A sweet sensation such as honey can allay nausea by disrupting sensation perception. A sorbet or ice pop can suppress the urge as well – the cold mouth feeling brings a competing message and can hack into the vagus nerve and reset the body/brain perception. Try sipping some iced water or iced green tea. Coconut water has all the electrolytes the body needs to replenish hydration and level out recovery. Lemon juice is a traditional cure.

The Benefit of Deep Breathing

When you breathe deeply, you not only fill your lungs but also bring oxygen into the abdomen, and the filling and releasing action (combined with the oxygen flush) facilitates a release and relaxation effect upon abdominal muscles and the diaphragm. This can dramatically reduce stomach tension and alleviate feelings of nausea. It can also suppress the urge to vomit and the spasms that assist it.

Method

Begin by inhaling slowly, through the nose – deep into the chest – then exhale normally from your mouth. Next time breathe deeper – into the abdomen – let your belly protrude and fill with air. Exhale gently through your mouth. Now inhale as much air as you can, filling your belly and lungs to capacity – hold a moment – now slowly exhale through the mouth – slow and steady, let the air out of the tyre. Repeat for a few cycles.

Different Pressure

Try a little acupressure. Nei Kuan or the P6 acupressure point is located three finger-widths below your wrist, thumb side, between the two central tendons. It is the point that calms anxiety and decreases nausea and vomiting.

Method

Locate the acupressure point and apply gentle pressure with the thumb of your other hand for 3 minutes. Then swivel or rock your thumb to massage the spot for a further 2 minutes. Take a break for a few moments and repeat the cycles until your nausea subsides.

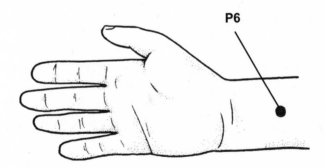

NEURALGIA

Neuralgia is a medical term that defines any pain originating from a nerve, most often manifesting as a stabbing, sharp or burning pain. A lot of pain is 'referred' and this is more than true with neuralgia – meaning while you experience it in your foot its source may be a trapped nerve in your vertebrae, as with sciatica (see page 215). Trigeminal neuralgia affects one side of the face and is often triggered by a blood vessel pressing down on the trigeminal nerve. Glossopharyngeal neuralgia can strike not only the throat and tongue, but also be 'referred' to the ear or neck – occasioned by pressure or injury to the glossopharyngeal nerve. Analgesics can help but the emphasis should be on nerve health. When it comes to nervine herbs there are two paths and both get you there. Firstly nervine tonics, aka trophorestoratives, which build up nerve health and function, and secondly nervine relaxants that soothe nerve endings and calm signalling.

Garden treatments

Gamma-linolenic acid (GLA) is an anti-inflammatory agent that also helps with pain sensitivity and pain perception – it is in borage oil and evening primrose oil. Mint, in culinary terms, suppresses neuralgia but in topical rubs it can lessen pain signals by disrupting perception with its cool sensation. Analgesic herbs such as lavender, rosemary, eucalyptus and chamomile in essential or sun-infused oil form can also be beneficial in topical applications at the area of the pain. Meadowsweet tea is pain relieving. Potent nervine tonic herbs include borage and St John's wort, while relaxants (some are also adaptogens so have the extra benefit of lowering stress levels) include lavender, lemon balm, chamomile, hops, skullcap and passionflower. Lemon balm is particularly effective for neuralgia.

Kitchen support

Eating chillies depletes substance P – the signal system of pain. Celery has phytochemicals that soothe neuralgic pain signals – so take as you like in soup, juiced, braised or in Waldorf salad. Oats are nervine. Dairy and other foods with calcium and magnesium can relax affected muscles and take the pressure off nerve endings. B vitamins, especially B1, B2 and biotin, support nerve function and are nervine in nature – oats, mushrooms, avocados, sunflower seeds and Swiss chard all contain a good supply. Almonds, berries and bananas contain biotin and also have analgesic and sedative properties. Vitamin E from avocados, seeds, nuts, wholegrains and vegetable oils (particularly wheatgerm and sunflower oil) is essential for nerve health and recovery. Omega-3 oils are involved in the manufacture of GLA – great for nerve health and to alleviate your pain.

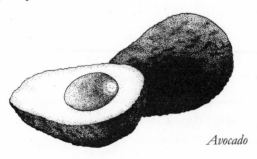

Avocado

GLA-D Tidings Hot Sauce (with GLA and vitamin D)

For pain relief and mood elevation.

Ingredients

- 2 red bell peppers
- 1 tablespoon olive oil
- 2 large tomatoes
- 50g chillies (mild to medium are good for this, but if you like it hot go for it)
- 4 cloves garlic
- 2 leaves lemon balm
- 1 tablespoon grated ginger
- 10fl oz red wine vinegar
- 1 tablespoon salt
- 5 tablespoons sugar
- 3 tablespoons honey
- 2 tablespoons evening primrose or borage oil
- 1 teaspoon coconut oil

Method

Halve and deseed the bell peppers, grease with olive oil and roast in the oven at a high heat until the skin blackens and blisters a bit and can be removed. Meanwhile core and roughly chop the tomatoes, slice and deseed the chillies, peel the garlic and shred the lemon balm. Bring all of these, plus the ginger, to a boil in the vinegar and salt and simmer for 10 minutes. Add a dash of water if the liquid is evaporating too quickly. Add the sugar and stir until it dissolves. Again add a dash of water if required. Roughly chop the skinned peppers and add to a blender, then pour in the cooked chilli mix and purée. Finally, add the honey, borage or evening primrose oil and the coconut oil and blitz again. Decant to a storage container and enjoy. This keeps best in the fridge – for a week plus – but it won't last that long once you have it on chips or some suitably healthy alternative.

PREMENSTRUAL SYNDROME (PMS)

PMS is linked to hormonal fluxes and affects around 75 per cent of menstruating women, with varying intensity and divergence in symptomatic experience. Symptoms commence anywhere from five to eleven days before menstruation and for the most part dissipate once menstruation begins – or are integrated or masked by the symptoms of period pains (see page 183). Symptoms of PMS include cramping (see page 195), bloating (see page 102), tender breasts, headaches (see page 149), anxiety (see page 237), depression or sadness, irritability, insomnia (see page 178), sensitivity to light or sound, acne, food cravings, diarrhoea (see page 95) or constipation (see page 75).

Garden treatments

A little sunshine works wonders, as it raises our capacity to synthesise vitamin D into serotonin and there is a connection between low serotonin levels and PMS. Plant any type of plant – there is a bacterium in soil that, on contact with skin, causes the brain to produce more serotonin. When it comes to harvesting, try picking some diuretics such as cranberries, blue cohosh, burdock, fennel, horsetail, nettle, parsley and meadowsweet – they can help to ease both bloating and water retention. Note that most diuretics remove not just fluids from the body but also some vitamins and minerals – coconut water replaces any lost electrolytes and dandelion tea is diuretic without the potassium flushing.

Many of the diuretics I mention here have extra value in treating PMS. Cranberries are not only anti-inflammatory but also help to reduce prostaglandins and contain potassium and magnesium, which ease cramping. Blue cohosh is antispasmodic and analgesic. Black cohosh is a phytoestrogen that lessens progesterone and so triggers a hormonal rebalance. Burdock is detoxing and packed with vitamin B6, which regulates your internal clock for a better night's sleep and endorphin release, with a knock-on effect on your mood and well-being. Fennel is also antispasmodic. Horsetail and nettle supply calcium and other nutrients lost during periods. Parsley is a hormone balancer and meadowsweet is analgesic.

Chaste tree has a long history in balancing female hormones and is also used for acne, headaches and inflammation, nausea, diarrhoea, muscle aches and joint pain. The GLA in borage oil and evening primrose oil can help to alleviate breast pain and may actually remedy all ancillary symptoms of PMS. The liver is vital to clearing excess oestrogen so garden hepatics are a good option – try dandelion, goldenseal, milk thistle or St John's wort.

Kitchen support

Drinking plenty of fluids will ease abdominal bloating while foods rich in vitamin B6 (avocados, pistachio nuts, sunflower seeds), folic acid (lentils, spinach, avocados), calcium (mozzarella, tofu, yoghurt) and magnesium (lentils, brown rice, pumpkin seeds) help reduce both cramping and mood swings. Hepatic supportive foods include apples, beetroot, garlic, horseradish, olive oil, parsley, broccoli, brown rice, Brussels sprouts, cabbage, carrots, oat bran, spinach and tomatoes.

Burdock, Carrot and Parsley Broth

Ingredients
- A piece of burdock root (10–15cms or so)
- 4 cups water
- 1 carrot
- 1 tablespoon chopped parsley
- Optional – salt and pepper to taste

Method
Peel the burdock root, soak it in water for 15 minutes, rinse it off, and cut it into coins of approximately 1cm in length. Add to a saucepan with the water and bring to a boil. Boil for 5 minutes, then simmer for 20. Meanwhile peel and wash the carrot and cut into coins also. Wash and finely chop the parsley. Add the carrots and parsley to the pot at the end of the burdock's simmering time. Simmer for a further 30 minutes or until the burdock and carrot coins are soft. I like the look of this chunky broth and generally just season and serve. You can of course purée to a soup and add a swirl of cream.

SCIATICA AND PIRIFORMIS SYNDROME

Sciatica is a condition of radiating pain caused by agitation or compression of the sciatic nerve – the longest nerve in your body – running from the pelvis, down both legs to your feet. Sometimes a slipped disc is the contributing factor. Most herniated disks resolve themselves within about six weeks. Pain relief is the first port of call but, whether acute or persistent, minimising sciatic incidences necessitates a look at better posture and engaging with gentle regular exercise to improve flexibility.

Piriformis syndrome is a slightly rarer type of sciatica and involves a buttock muscle called the piriformis pinching or pushing against the sciatic nerve. Anti-inflammatories are excellent treatment for this, but are also central to the treatment of standard sciatica.

Garden treatments

St John's wort has a long history of use to treat nerve pain. Beyond being anti-inflammatory and slightly analgesic, it is chosen for its ability to assist regeneration of nerve tissue. As well as the internal use of the herb, St John's wort oil is a topical treatment for

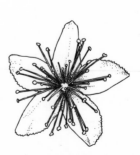

St John's wort

inflammation too. A superior pain liniment can be made with wintergreen. It contains plenty of methyl salicylate – as seen in the ingredients list of many over-the-counter neuromuscular pain relief treatments and products for inflammation reduction. Horse chestnut extract is beneficial for lower and sacroiliac pain – modify the horse chestnut gel (see page 252) with several pinches of turmeric, fennel and chilli powder to yield a refreshing and pain-desensitising rub. There are many garden-sourced anti-inflammatories, but chamomile has a particular affinity with the sciatic nerve (with the benefit of delivering the potent pain reliever bisabolol).

Kitchen support

Many common spices, such as ginger, have anti-inflammatory properties, but both garlic and turmeric directly diminish the body's supply of enzymes that fuel the inflammation response. When it comes to fruits and veg many are natural anti-inflammatories thanks to their carotenoid content, but those rich in a carotenoid called beta-cryptoxanthin (packed into orange-coloured fruits and vegetables) are more pronounced in their anti-inflammatory effect – have sweet potato and carrots for dinner, cantaloupe and orange juice for breakfast.

Posture Exercise

The yoga pose known as *Supta Padangusthasana* can help realign and strengthen your lower back's muscular system and alleviate sciatica complications; it also specifically targets and loosens piriformis muscles.

Method

- Sit flat and breathe for a moment to centre yourself.
- Loop a long belt or yoga strap over the ball of your foot.
- Lie flat on your back keeping hold of the strap.
- Holding the strap and tightening your grip, allow your leg to rise towards the sky.
- As you stretch the leg upwards, keep your foot flexed and your buttocks pressed to the floor.

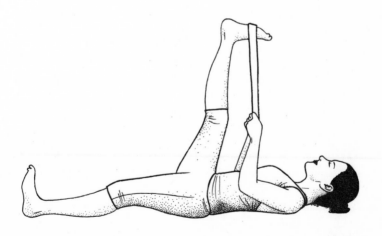

- Hold the pose and count through ten breaths.
- Now slowly bend the knee towards your chest, loosen your grip and then let your leg lower to the floor.
- Pause a moment then repeat the process with the other leg.
- Do this three to five times for each leg; increase repetitions for each session – next time try five to seven, then seven to ten.
- Doing these exercises two or three times a week will strengthen what needs strengthening and loosen what needs opening up.

SINUSITIS

Sinusitis is an inflammatory condition caused by a viral or bacterial infection or a triggering allergen affecting the lining of the sinuses and presenting as a blocked or runny nose. Ancillary symptoms can include high temperature, headache (see page 149) and facial pain. Sinusitis is often considered either *acute* or *chronic*. *Acute* develops quickly over a period of a few days and clears within weeks. *Chronic* can persist for several months.

We each have four pairs of sinuses, one behind the forehead, one behind the eyes, one behind the cheekbones and one at either side of the bridge of the nose. The largest ones, those behind the cheekbones, are most commonly affected.

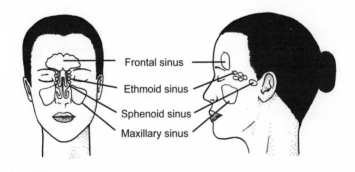

Frontal sinus
Ethmoid sinus
Sphenoid sinus
Maxillary sinus

Garden treatment

Nettles have antihistamine action to alleviate sinus congestion. Inhalations of mint are decongestant; inhalations of lavender, thyme or eucalyptus are anti-catarrhal and somewhat antispasmodic. See also pages 60–1 for decongesting herbs. Sinusitis is an inflammatory condition so while antihistamines tackle the allergic reaction, try basil, rosemary, parsley, St John's wort or mint to take down the swelling.

Kitchen support

Both wasabi and horseradish are traditional remedies for sinus problems but their teary-eyed strength can be a bit much for some. If so, try fruit – grapefruit helps reduce salt build-up in the body and so eases swelling, but it also naturally speeds up the elimination of thick mucus. Citrus fruits full of vitamin C tackle toxins and decrease inflammation reactions. Pineapples are packed with proteolytic enzymes that break down and neutralise bradykinins and eicosanoids – the biochemical building blocks of inflammation. Try a pineapple, mango and orange sorbet or smoothie.

Dairy, sugar and processed foods can prolong sinus inflammation so dietary changes around flare-ups can speed the healing process. Anti-inflammatory herbs include turmeric, cayenne, ginger, cloves, cinnamon, rosemary and sage. Orange foods rich in vitamin A or beta-carotene help with the production of mucopolysaccharide, the vital protective barrier component of the mucous membranes.

Saline Nasal Rinse

Ingredients
- Non-iodised salt
- Baking soda
- Still water

Method
Stir 2 teaspoons of non-iodised salt and 1 teaspoon of baking soda into 1 pint of distilled or sterile/post-boiled water. Decant to a sterilised bottle with a lid and store at room temperature. Best used within two weeks. Shake well before use.

How to use: a bulb syringe or neti pot is helpful in the application of saline solution. Position yourself with your head over a sink and tilted to one side. Disperse or pour the saline solution directly into the upper nostril – the angle of your head will allow the solution to pass through your nasal cavity and run out the other nostril. Some will go down the back of your throat – you can spit that out. Now gently blow your nose to clear the nasal passages of solution and any loosened catarrh. Tilt your head in the opposite direction and apply to the other nostril.

Seasonal Nettle, Basil and Parsley Pesto

This brings some savoury antihistamine and anti-inflammatory action.

Ingredients

- ¾ cup pine nuts
- 2 cups nettle leaves
- ½ cup basil
- ⅓ cup parsley
- 5 garlic cloves
- ¾ cup grated hard cheese (traditionally pecorino or parmesan)
- ½ cup olive oil
- 1 teaspoon honey
- Pinch of salt

Method

Heat a skillet and lightly toast the pine nuts. Blanch the nettles in boiling water or wilt on a hot skillet to remove the sting histamines. Add all the ingredients to a blender and blitz to the consistency you prefer – textured, smooth or outright creamy. Decant to a storage container and pour a glug of olive oil on the top to seal in freshness. Seal and store in the fridge – this will typically keep for three weeks.

SORE THROAT

Sore throats can manifest as an individual ailment or arise in conjunction with the common cold (see page 64), flu (see page 67), seasonal allergies (see page 145), etc.

Viral: it is estimated that almost 90 per cent of sore throats are viral. Antibiotics don't work against viruses.

Bacterial: the most common bacterial infection of the throat is *Streptococcus*, thus the term strep throat. Strep throat is often accompanied by fever, enlarged lymph nodes and visible white patches in your throat.

Allergic: a sore throat can be one of the symptoms of hay fever or allergic rhinitis and treating the underlying condition in conjunction with alleviation of the sore throat is best practice.

Garden treatments

Agrimony in tea or tincture form is astringent and acts against sore throats – as a gargle, combine with thyme or mint to kill off triggering microbes. Echinacea is both antiviral and antibacterial, as is thyme – both these herbs can be made into teas, tinctures, syrups and even ice pops or slush puppies to let the chill factor soothe and relieve. Both marshmallow root and liquorice root contain plenty of mucilage, which soothes mucous membranes in the throat and coats the lining against further irritation.

Traditionally tinctures of barberry protect the lining of the throat and attack viral and bacterial infections (dosage is generally 15 or so drops in ¼ cup of water, three times daily for a week). Rosemary or mint gargles are excellent to de-inflame and pack an antimicrobial punch.

Kitchen support

One of the simplest cures is to gargle with warm salty water (1 teaspoon of salt to half a cup of room temperature – or just above – water). Sea or table, the salt decreases bacteria and helps to draw toxins from swollen cells and decrease inflammation. Many swear by a warm infusion of lemon and honey but also honey direct from a spoon or just slightly diluted with some herbal tea imparts antimicrobial action and is soothing to gritty or sharp sore throats. The high acidity level of apple cider vinegar can help kill bacteria infecting your throat if you gargle with it – it's OK to swallow too, as it also helps to boost your immune system. You can dilute a tablespoon in half a cup of water if straight is too strong for you.

Munching raw garlic is remedial to all three types of sore throat and the allicin compounds not only kill off the germs but also help decrease pain and irritation. While you're about it, eating some horseradish will treat a sore throat while also assisting with upper respiratory tract infections and excess mucus. Clove tea, more often utilised to numb the pain of sore teeth, contains eugenol, which will also slightly numb the throat – I use clove as a ground spice in honey whenever I get a sore throat.

Strawberry and Lime Sugar-Free Vitamin C Ice Lolly

A raw food answer to a raw throat. Depending on the size of the moulds it will deliver four to six ice pops.

Ingredients
- 1lb ripe fresh strawberries
- 2 tablespoons lime juice
- Moulds and ice-pop sticks

Method
Wash and hull the strawberries; add to a blender with the lime juice and purée. Decant to moulds; place in the freezer for 4 hours or until fully frozen. To remove from the mould in one smooth move, simply dip the bottom of the mould in warm water for 10–15 seconds.

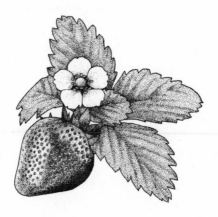

LARYNGITIS

Laryngitis is a viral or bacterial infection of the respiratory tract – specifically triggering inflammation of the mucous membrane lining of the larynx (voice box). It presents as hoarseness and in extreme cases as a temporary loss of speech. Your natural inclination may be to whisper but whispering actually puts a greater strain on the vocal cords than attempting to speak as normal. It can last up to several weeks and, while there is no cure (other than the waiting game), there is relief.

Garden treatments

Steam inhalations are very beneficial and we can further medicate that steam with a judicious application of garden herbs and medicinal plants. Try adding a few leaves of thyme, lavender or rosemary to a basin of hot water and use a towel over your head, with your head over the basin, to make a steam tent – breathe as normal inside it. Soothing gargles can also be made from cooled infusions or decoctions of eucalyptus, thyme, mint, chamomile, goldenrod, meadowsweet and marshmallow foliage. Mullein has a history as a demulcent and barberry is effective against infection of the respiratory tract.

Kitchen support

Keep hydrated. Those herbal gargles make nice herbal teas too. Honey is a soother and antimicrobial. Honey and lemon work a treat. Both garlic and ginger raise white blood cells and treat infection.

Honey and Lemonicious Lozenges

Soreness soothers with antimicrobial action.

Ingredients
- 5 leaves lemon balm
- 2 tablespoons lemon juice
- 85g sugar
- 2 tablespoons water
- 85g honey
- Cornflour

Method
Purée the lemon balm with 1 tablespoon of lemon juice. Add the sugar, water and the other tablespoon of lemon juice to a saucepan and bring to the boil, stirring constantly. When the sugar fully dissolves, stir in the lemon balm purée and then add the honey – bring to boiling point and remove from the heat. The mixture will thicken as it cools. Spread out a sheet of parchment paper or prepare a silicone mould and dust with a little cornflour. Using a teaspoon, make coin shapes on the parchment paper or fill the moulds. Let the lozenges fully cool and set. Dust the tops with cornflour. Store in an airtight container and use as required. These will keep in a dry, cool location for many weeks.

TONSILLITIS

Your tonsils are part of your lymphatic system. Tonsillitis is a bacterial infection, often caused by streptococcus, that results in sore throat sensations with pain on swallowing, enlarged glands and sometimes an elevated temperature. Referred pain to the ear can accompany the infection and also fatigue (see page 123), vomiting (see page 204) and stomach ache.

Garden treatments

Thyme or echinacea (or both combined) are excellent as immune-boosting teas and antibacterial gargles. Other antibacterial and soothing herbs for sore throats can be found on pages 223–4, but a great approach is to think about herbs that boost the lymphatic system and strengthen it against attack. Cleavers in cool infused water or as a tea, a smoothie or in tincture form activates lymphatic drainage. Other lymph detoxifiers (or herbs with lymphagogue action) include red clover, milk thistle, devil's claw, goldenseal, calendula, aloe vera, bloodroot, burdock and dandelion root. Gargles of cooled decoctions of lovage root can help – combine with thyme, mint or angelica leaf for anti-inflammatory and antimicrobial action.

Kitchen support

Honey is soothing and antimicrobial. Strengthen your immune system with garlic, which is also antibacterial. You might not feel like eating much so have a half-day fast (but keep hydrated) then have a smoothie of raw fruit – the fruit enzymes and fruit acids are natural lymph-system cleansers, boosted by being consumed on an empty stomach.

Infused Cleaver Water

This is an excellent detoxing beverage.

Method
Pick a stalk (with leaves), rinse under a tap and add to a tall glass of water, or add several stalks to a jug. Chill in the fridge for 2 hours. Remove the cleaver or keep as a garnish and ongoing infusion. Sip and enjoy.

Pitcher Chiller

An antimicrobial, lymph-cleansing and anti-inflammatory drink.

Ingredients
- 2 tablespoons milk thistle tea
- 2 tablespoons lemon thyme tea (or other herbal tea of choice)
- 2 tablespoons honey
- 1 cup lime juice
- 1 cup lemon juice

Method
Put 2 tablespoons of each tea into a teapot with 2 cups of boiling water, then stir in the honey until it dissolves. Allow to infuse for 20 minutes, then add the liquid to a pitcher with the juices and chill for 2 hours before sipping throughout the rest of the day.

STOMACH UPSETS – GASTROENTERITIS AND FOOD POISONING

These upsets can occasion diarrhoea (see page 95) and vomiting (see page 204). They are not minor upsets such as cramp or bloating (see page 102), but infections of the stomach and often bowel.

GASTROENTERITIS

Often referred to as gastric flu, this is most often caused by a viral or bacterial infection of the stomach and bowel. Viral infection is most frequently caused by a rotavirus or norovirus (see winter vomiting bug, page 266), while bacterial infection is commonly a case of food poisoning (see page 233), contaminated water (transmitting more often a parasitic rather than bacterial infection) or an ingested pathogen. Symptoms include stomach upset, queasiness, recurrent episodes of diarrhoea (generally three or more within a twenty-four-hour period), nausea and vomiting (see page 204).

Garden treatments

While plants such as petasites have a history of antispasmodic action, one can easily avail of garden mint or peppermint tea, which not only are antispasmodic but also can decrease bacterial complications. Meadowsweet tea is a natural aspirin – so pain relieving – and helps to reduce sensations of nausea. It is also effective at soothing inflamed mucous membranes within the stomach and gastrointestinal tract. Herbs to boost the immune system include garlic, liquorice, ginger, ginseng and thyme.

Kitchen support

When I was a child arrowroot biscuits were a part of my mother's medicinal canon but the powder form – a culinary thickening agent made from 100 per cent arrowroot (which, as the name suggests, was formerly used to cure arrow wounds) is soothing on the digestive tract and intestines. Its starch and fibre work on the lower bowel and it has good levels of B vitamins essential for convalescence. Make up as a warm drink by adding hot milk or hot water, or add to soup.

There are many culinary herbs with antispasmodic properties, not least basil and oregano. Thyme and garlic can kill stomach bugs while simultaneously boosting immune-system response.

You might not feel like a meal but you need to eat and drink to keep energy levels up and to maintain nutrition in a steady supply. A light meal will do – think of easy to digest foods, but not dairy fats such as cheese, or spicy or sugary foods that can aggravate the lining of your stomach. There is merit in a BRAT diet – that is bananas, rice, apple sauce and toast. It doesn't all have to be on the same plate but apple sauce on toast is lovely and bananas in rice is like a pudding – so you can mix it up. These four give a bit of energy but place no strain on the system.

A Soothie Smoothie for Tricky Tums in Recovery

Ripe bananas are a constipant and restorative. Honey supplies energy and is antibacterial and antiviral, while live yoghurt boosts the immune system and soothes the digestive tract.

Method

To a cup of yoghurt add 1 ripe banana and 1 teaspoon of honey. Blitz and enjoy chilled.

Pepperminty Jelly

An alternative to mint tea but with all the cramp-busting and bactericidal properties intact. Plus it's a great way to ease back into swallowing food.

Method

Per cup-quantity required, blitz 10 peppermint leaves in a cup of boiling water (blitzing rather than simply infusing keeps more constituents in the final product). Then, to set, add 1 teaspoon of agar powder. Allow to set with the bits in. Enjoy. Other setting agents – carrageen moss, gelatine or veg gel crystals – work equally well.

FOOD POISONING

This is contracted from eating food contaminated with harmful bacteria. It manifests as diarrhoea (see page 95), abdominal cramps and vomiting (see page 204), the combination of which can bring about dehydration and headaches (see page 149). Fever (see page 133) accompanies some instances depending on the pathogen. Food-poisoning-like symptoms can also be caused by liver and gastric viruses (hepatitis A), disease and parasites. Of the more than 250 different pathogens that can cause food poisoning, the most common are the infectious bacterial implications of *Campylobacter, Clostridium perfringens, E. coli, Salmonella* or a norovirus.

- **Campylobacter** infection results in cramps, fever, vomiting and diarrhoea, which may be bloody. It has an incubation period of 2–5 days and illness of 2–10 days. It's commonly contracted from raw/undercooked poultry, unpasteurised milk and contaminated water.

- **Clostridium perfringens** presents as diarrhoea and abdominal cramps (neither fever nor vomiting are present); it may persist for 1–2 weeks. The incubation period is 6–24 hours. Contraction is via meat, reheated leftovers and long-standing 'warm' food.

- **E. coli** is a bacterium that naturally lives in the intestines of humans and animals. It can enter the food chain through unhygienic/faecal contamination but also via raw milk and some raw foods. The incubation is 1–10 days with illness of 5–10 days. It presents as severe diarrhoea (often

233

bloody) with intense abdominal pain and vomiting. Fever is slight if present at all.

- **Salmonella** is associated with unpasteurised milk, raw or lightly cooked eggs, undercooked poultry and meats. It has an incubation period of 12–72 hours with symptoms lasting 4–7 days. It presents classically with abdominal cramps, diarrhoea, fever and vomiting.

- **Norovirus** – see winter vomiting bug (see page 266).

Garden treatments

Garden-sourced antibiotics to tackle the infection include chamomile, thyme, yellow dock, lavender, St John's wort, goldenseal and red clover. Any immunity boosters such as echinacea or thyme or health store pau d'arco will help. Antispasmodics can address cramp – try cramp bark, catmint, chamomile, liquorice, peppermint and black cohosh. Marshmallow and slippery elm both have soothing and regenerating effects upon the lining of the stomach. Echinacea is a great support as it contains many helpful biochemicals. These include echinacein, which neutralises hyaluronidase – a tissue-dissolving enzyme produced by bacteria to help with bacterial proliferation. Another, called echinacoside, is a powerful antibiotic capable of destroying or limiting a broad range of bacteria, fungi and protozoa and also viruses.

Kitchen support

Dehydration is significant, so drink water, tea, juice, etc. to keep hydrated. Artichoke is hepatic protective (strengthens and detoxifies the liver). It is used in herbal treatments for a range of digestive disorders, including many of the symptoms of food poisoning, and also exhibits antimicrobial activities useful in diminishing bacterial infection. Raw cabbage, cabbage juice and fermented cabbage combat *H. pylori, Salmonella* and other bacterial triggers of this condition. Raw cabbage is high in glutamine, an amino acid essential for intestinal health and to help recovery. Garlic contains sulphur compounds that undermine bacterial proliferation. Its allicin is certainly one of its most potent compounds and exerts powerful antimicrobial activities within the gut and bloodstream. Allicin is very effective against *E. coli* and the other agents of this condition. It also exhibits anti-parasitic and antiviral activities.

Honey, cloves, cinnamon and mustard are antibacterial and germicidal. Thyme, basil and sage are antispasmodic and immunostimulant. Coconut oil contains lauric acid which, when ingested, is converted to monolaurin, a rather potent monoglyceride compound which injures the lipid membrane structures of fungi, bacteria and viruses. You could eat a spoonful daily direct from the spoon, or add it into cooking.

Clover and Echinacea Leaf Tea

The phytochemicals and polysaccharides in the aerial parts of echinacea are better than the root parts to stimulate the immune system. Red clover is a natural antibiotic.

Method

To a cup of boiling water add a teaspoon of the chopped foliage of both plants and let them infuse for 10 minutes. Sweetening with honey is fine and even antimicrobial, but avoid sugar or artificial sweeteners.

Raw Red Cabbage Slaw

Ingredients

- ½ carrot
- ¼ head red cabbage
- 1 scallion
- 1 teaspoon coconut oil, melted
- 1 tablespoon apple cider vinegar
- 1 tablespoon mustard
- 2 tablespoons sour cream
- 3 tablespoons lemon or lime juice
- A pinch of salt

Method

Peel, wash and julienne or grate the carrot. Wash and shred the cabbage. Dice the scallion. Place the vegetables in a bowl and mix. Add the remaining ingredients and fold together well. Chill to serve.

STRESS AND ANXIETY

Stress is often seen as a state of mind but it is physical too and is both the mind's and the body's natural reaction to a perceived or real threat or danger. Stress is often seen as a pressure exerted by an external source – a work deadline, a sick child, a bill to be paid, etc. Often it is a pressure we put on ourselves, by overextending ourselves or biting off more than we can chew. Yes, there is a benefit in easing up, but understanding stress can help lessen its ability to grip us psychologically. Stress is not abstract: it is a fundamental part of the workings of the human machine. Stress and all its responses, including anxiety, panic, insomnia (see page 178) and appetite changes, are the consequence of our inherent 'fight or flight' response. We evolved this mechanism to pre-emptively release hormones such as adrenaline and corticosteroids, so that if the rustle behind us turns out to be a tiger we get enough of a surge to punch it on the nose or run away from it. These are the two best natural survival responses – get the threat out of the way or get the hell out of its way. But in the modern world how do you punch away or run off excess hormones when it's only somebody in your parking space or the thousandth menu in the letter box this week – we still get the hit of hormones pushing all our buttons but we have no way to use them up. We carry this hit to the next pushed button and each pushed button in a given day has more biochemical impact.

So we need to employ some strategies to escape our reactions to perceived threats or situations that we connect with danger or anger. Mindfulness is excellent, as is some physical action – if you miss your train, instead of having a tantrum do a few star jumps or some skipping on the spot: it will work *and* keep you limber. A sense of humour is key, as it activates happiness, which is the antidote to stress hormones. Of course chemical constituents in food and plants can counter the surges and ease the system too. See also fatigue (page 123) and insomnia (page 178).

Garden treatments

Prescribed anti-anxiety pharmaceuticals target gamma-amino-butyric acid (GABA) receptors in the brain to influence neural signalling and calm the central nervous system – thus providing a more tranquil experience. Chamomile, parsley, thyme, yarrow, vervain and other herbs and foods with apigenin have similar GABA-influencing properties. Chamomile is equally effective in the form of a natural soothing beverage or an aroma. It also significantly influences or triggers monoamine neurotransmitters – which include serotonin and dopamine, the 'happy' hormones. Likewise as a tea, culinary herb or aroma, lavender has the ability to neutralise stress thoughts and effect a calm response. Infusions of lemon balm foliage are packed with the phytochemical terpene that reduces stress responses and promotes calm, as does valerian tea.

Passionflower is another powerful anxiolytic (reduces anxiety and stress responses) and has a long herbal tradition in treating anxiety, apprehension and excitability – the flowers, leaves and stems of the plant yield a slightly sedative tea; capsules of the herb are readily available. Similarly, infusions of evening primrose flowers are reputed to reduce mental stress; the calming neurotransmitter support of gamma-linolenic acid in evening primrose oil is beneficial also and easily sourced in a local health store. The roots of rhodiola are considered an adaptogen and thus help the system cope more effectively with mental, physical, biochemical and even environmental stresses. Basil is also adaptogenic, as are white mulberry, sea buckthorn and schizandra berries. At the extreme end of the anxiety spectrum St John's wort has a long history of use as a regenerative nervine for both neurologic and psychiatric disorders. Hyssop tea is sedative.

Kitchen support

Comfort eating long term can lead to obesity, but sometimes a little comfort food makes a suitable medicine for a bad day. I'm not saying dial for a ten-thousand-calorie takeaway, but a little tryptophan is not bad. Tryptophan is an essential amino acid contained in milk, cheese, bananas and other sources of protein. It regulates sleep and releases serotonin, a hormone which could be regarded as the neurotransmitter of well-being and psychological stability. 5-HTP found in potatoes supports serotonin production and efficacy. Oats are naturally nervine and their B vitamins are beneficial to stabilising mood – make porridge or flapjacks (see page 269).

Apigenin is an amazing bioflavonoid compound for general health and lauded for its anticancer properties, but it is also an anxiolytic compound working directly on brain chemistry and signalling pathways to make us feel better and more relaxed. It is abundant in parsley, basil, tarragon, coriander, oregano, celery, onions, grapefruit, oranges and the fruits of passionflowers. It is also in beer and red wine, which is perhaps why so many people self-medicate that way – but why have a hangover when a diet of fruits and veg will energise your physical self and that, in itself, energises your psychological self too?

Clementine, Passionfruit and Chamomile Coulis

Drizzle over cereals, fold into natural yoghurt or add to sparkling water as a cordial.

Ingredients

- 1 teaspoon chopped chamomile
- 1 cup boiling water
- 1 cup sugar
- ½ cup honey
- 1 cup passionfruit pulp (approximately 6–8 fruits)
- Juice and flesh of 2 clementines
- Juice of 2 lemons
- 1 teaspoon tartaric acid

Method

Make a cup of chamomile tea. Strain the solids from the tea and add the liquid and the sugar to a saucepan. Bring to the boil, stirring constantly until fully dissolved. Remove from the heat and add the honey – stirring well. Add the passionfruit pulp to the saucepan along with the lemon and clementine juice. Add the flesh of the clementines and the tartaric acid, bring back to the boil and reduce for 3 minutes, constantly stirring. Let it sit off the heat, covered, for 10 minutes. Push through a sieve to strain out the seeds and clementine flesh and pour the strained mixture into a clean bottle. This will store in the refrigerator for three weeks.

Bath Bliss Blitz

Time out is a short-term cure. But notching up positive moments is the long-term cure.

Ingredients
- 5 tablespoons chopped mint
- 5 tablespoons chopped lemon balm
- 5 tablespoons chopped lavender
- 3 tablespoons Epsom salt
- 1 tablespoon sea salt
- 2 teaspoons powdered mustard
- 2 cups Castile or other liquid soap

Method
Add all the ingredients to a blender and blitz to a smooth pulp. Decant to a storage container. Use a couple of tablespoons at a time as a bath additive to relax the mind and invigorate the body.

TOOTHACHE AND TOOTH DECAY

There are home cures to dull the pain; there are ones to fight the infection at source or boost the immune system. But some teeth need filling or removing – so a dentist's appointment is the best course of action. That said, all the remedies here will help alleviate symptoms and, if used early enough, prevent caries.

Garden treatment

Mint, thyme and rosemary make great antimicrobial rinses – all three are anti-inflammatory and slightly analgesic too. Natural aspirin is found in meadowsweet tea and willow leaf tea. Chewing willow bark was the original dental pain relief. Walking barefoot in the garden is a flip-switch to release and increase antioxidant and anti-inflammatory action within your body. Some acupressure points useful while out in the fresh air include Tai Xi or Nei Ting on the feet, He Gu on the hand or Jia Che on the jaw. Activate them by applying gentle pressure to the point/position of a meridian line – it's a sort of touch version of acupuncture.

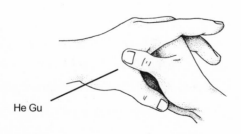

He Gu

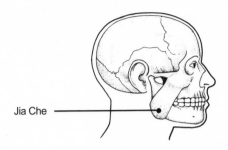

Jia Che

Kitchen support

Cloves and olive oil have anaesthetising principles, so a paste made of both can numb the pain. Rinsing with salt water can reduce inflammation and infection. As salt is antibacterial, it helps to sterilise the mouth and its osmotic action pulls toxins from the gum line of the affected tooth. Cinnamon is also antibacterial. You know what you shouldn't be eating, so avoid sugar – it is not only harmful to tooth enamel but also slows your immune system.

Top tip

Facts to brush up on. The right toothbrush has handles and bristles with angles, which are good, but really it's all about the stiffness of the bristle – sturdy enough to lift off plaque but not so hard as to be abrasive on teeth or aggravate gums. Current advice is to get a new brush every three or four months to avoid an ineffective brushing regime with worn down or frayed bristles. Try to remember a new one for each new season!

Sore Tooth Powder

All these ingredients have detoxing and antiseptic or antibacterial values.

Ingredients

- 1 tablespoon ground sea salt
- 1 teaspoon ground cloves
- 1 teaspoon ground cinnamon

Method

Mix all together. Store in a tin or jar. Simply dip a dry toothbrush into the mix and, sloshing a little saliva over your teeth, brush in a circular motion for 1–2 minutes, then rinse.

A Simple Salt-Water Rinse

References to the treating of gum disease and tooth decay with salt water appear as early as 2700 BCE in China's great healing systems and later in Greek and Roman materia medica. Salt is a natural disinfectant and kills the bacteria responsible for tooth decay and bad breath – it is also anti-inflammatory and somewhat analgesic to tooth pain. However, salty water is also acidic and so not for daily use.

Ingredients
- Salt – sea salt is best, but table salt can substitute on occasion
- Water – some tap water is fluoridated; some spring waters have calcium and other mineral traces beneficial to teeth

Method
Add 1 tablespoon of salt to a glass of water. Let the water warm to room temperature or add a little boiling water to help the salt dissolve and also to defer cold sensitivity. Rinse with it.

URINARY TRACT INFECTIONS – CYSTITIS AND BLADDER INFECTIONS

On one level cystitis and bladder infection are the same thing – infection of the urinary tract. Whatever way you look at it, it's a bacterial infection (often *E. coli* – see also page 233).

Cystitis is classically characterised by an increased frequency of urination – with urgency added to the need to empty the bladder. Urination can be painful and does not eliminate the need to go. Passed urine may look cloudy and be odorous and there may even be blood in the urine. Cystitis can include urethritis (an infection of the urethra) and acute pyelonephritis (infection of the kidney) as the infection-carrying urine is expelled with the contribution of kidneys, bladder and urethra.

Garden treatments

In traditional herbalism, horsetail tea is a genito-urinary astringent and lovage-root decoctions can treat urinary infections. In modern herbalism there are several ways to go – using diuretic herbs to flush out infection and reduce inflammation, availing of antispasmodics to diminish agitation or using urinary herbs to strengthen or soothe. Teas or culinary means are a great way to employ the actions of the various herbs. The better diuretics include agrimony, dandelion, yarrow, parsley, horsetail, woodruff, heartsease, meadowsweet, fennel, butcher's broom and hawthorn. Suitable antispasmodics include black cohosh, chamomile, hawthorn, juniper berries, catmint or cramp bark. You can take the antimicrobial route with thyme, lavender, goldenrod, goldenseal or uva ursi. Popular urinary demulcents such as couch grass, marshmallow and plantain can be used in moderation in a smoothie, as well as in a tea or tincture.

I favour urinary antiseptics – kill the bacteria, kill the condition. Heartsease tea, while diuretic, is also beneficial for treating painful urination. A plant chemical known as arbutin, a potent urinary-tract antiseptic and diuretic, can be found in a tea of bearberry leaves (contraindicated in pregnancy and not advised for longer than three weeks in other circumstances due to its high tannin content). It is also available from pears, cranberries and blueberries. My personal recommendations would include juniper berries because they are antibiotic, antispasmodic and diuretic – a three-hit wonder – and also yarrow tea (it increases urination and is antimicrobial, anti-inflammatory and antispasmodic) – a four-hit wonder. Uva ursi is a great urinary disinfectant but its effectiveness is diminished by the more easily sourced cranberry juice – so don't take both together.

Kitchen support

Our gut controls our immune system so use more natural yoghurt or acidophilus supplements to hurry up your own inherent natural antibacterial response. Barley water (see page 69) is beneficial – soothing to the system and restorative – but cranberry juice or indeed cranberry jelly is a natural urinary disinfectant – it produces hippuric acid in the urine, which increases acidity. This not only reduces bacteria but also prevents what's left from adhering to the walls of your bladder. Cranberries have antibacterial phytochemicals and their acidity kills the alkaline bacteria. Apple cider vinegar can help with that too, in the short term. Culinary diuretics include dill, fennel, horseradish, green tea, stevia, watercress and gooseberries. Culinary antispasmodics include sage, saffron, thyme, peppermint, rosemary and fennel bulb. In terms of antibacterial action, you won't go wrong with honey or garlic.

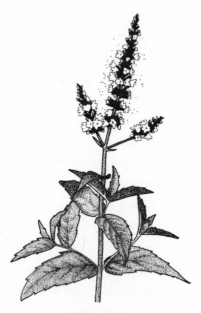

Peppermint

Sweet and Tangy Cranberry and Juniper Berry Compote

A tasty antimicrobial, anti-inflammatory and antispasmodic treat.

Ingredients

- 2 tablespoons juniper berries
- ½lb fresh cranberries (if dry, slightly less)
- ¼ cup cranberry juice
- ¼ cup orange juice
- 4 tablespoons sugar
- 2 tablespoons honey or orange marmalade
- Water

Method

Wash then crush the juniper berries with the flat side of a knife blade – place in a hot saucepan with a drop of water and cook for a minute. Next add the cranberries and the juices and bring to a boil. Simmer for 5 minutes, stirring regularly, then add the sugar and honey or marmalade. Keep stirring and simmer for a further 5 minutes or until thickening occurs. Remove from the heat and allow to cool completely before serving. Stores in the fridge for a week. Great on muesli, in natural yoghurt or, if so inclined, with meat dishes.

VENOUS INSUFFICIENCY AND VARICOSE VEINS

A circulatory issue called venous insufficiency, where the valves cannot move blood efficiently out of the veins back towards the heart, causes blood to pool and gather within the veins. This leads to swelling of the legs and ankles and over time the pooled blood and damage to cell walls can form varicose veins. Women seem to be more susceptible to chronic venous insufficiency than men, but it is by no means a gender-specific condition. So be it a noticeable blue line vein gaining prominence or an outright bunch of grapes, the treatments here address the insufficiency and the varicosity. Compression stockings work best but there is some good support too from the garden.

Garden treatments

Varicose veins can develop from standing in one place or sitting for long periods so pottering around the garden is a great way to get the circulation going. Take a barefoot walk across the lawn to boost your body's capacity to generate antioxidants, which is improved dramatically by grounding (making barefoot connection to the magnetic field of the earth). You can do this on the beach if you prefer to keep off the lawn. Butcher's broom inhibits both histamine and bradykinin reactions within the circulatory system, thus lessening their action of making the veins thin and permeable. St John's wort is anti-inflammatory and de-stresses veins (utilised topically and internally). Internally hawthorn strengthens capillaries; internally and externally, horse chestnuts do likewise.

Horse chestnuts are rich in saponins – one in particular, called escin, is both anti-inflammatory and vasoprotective. Tinctures and extracts have a long history as oral medications to recirculate trapped deoxygenated blood from bruises, haemorrhages and varicose veins. Escin is actually most beneficial in strengthening the walls of capillaries, veins and arteries – it effectively diminishes the presence of elastase and hyaluronidase, two enzymes that break down protein and contribute to venous insufficiency and those varicose veins. **Note of Caution** – part of its success is that the extract also thins the blood (technically by impairing the function and action of platelets), so be judicious with usage if on blood-thinning medication. The extract can be applied topically in lotion, gel, cream or compress formats.

Kitchen support

Avoid as much as possible sugary, fried, refined or processed foods which thicken blood and clog arteries with fats. Eat more fibre to cleanse your system and tone veins. Omega-3 fatty acids in tofu, walnuts and fish strengthen blood vessels. Soft fruits tone blood vessels. Garlic acts to strengthen them. Beetroot strengthens veins and tones capillaries. Pineapples, blackberries and cherries contain enzymes and phytochemicals beneficial in preventing and treating varicose vein symptoms. Cacao nibs contain epicatechin, a potent flavonol that improves blood vessel function; it also contains theobromine – a heart tonic. Swap the hot chocolate for some cacao.

Horse Chestnut Extract

An external rub to stimulate blood circulation and strengthen delicate blood vessels.

Method

In autumn gather some nuts and remove each nut from its spiny green case. Crack the shells and remove the meal. Place all the meal in a blender and cover completely with vodka. Blitz to a paste – add more vodka if the consistency is too thick.

Tinctures of horse chestnut for internal usage can be manufactured in the traditional way or bought standardised from health shops.

VERRUCAE

Verrucae are plantar warts that occur on the soles of feet and around toes and are caused by contact with the human papillomavirus (HPV) family. The virus is contagious and is often harboured in areas where bare feet and moist, damp environments connect, such as swimming pools, changing-room floors and communal shower areas. Verrucae are not so much harmful as uncomfortable, but scratching and picking at them will only spread them. Verrucae are identifiable as small cauliflower-type growths with tiny black dots visible.

Garden treatments

Most over-the-counter treatments contain salicylic acid (found in willow trees and meadowsweet), which, when applied topically to the wart, actively disintegrate the viral cells. Topically applied thyme oil and tea tree oil are great viral busters and disinfecting.

Kitchen support

Lemon juice is acidic enough to destroy some viral content in your skin cells but it may sting like an expletive of your choice. Oats and barley are said to draw toxins from the skin and an oat or barley footbath can rejuvenate the skin's own healing potential as the beta-glucan content is antimicrobial. You may prefer to keep the lemon juice for some honey and thyme tea to boost the immune system or eat some oats for the same purpose. Oats and barley are full of a beta-glucan which, beyond the antimicrobial factor, is a super antioxidant and a booster to the efficiency of other garden-grown antibiotics and antivirals. Garlic is topically antimicrobial and internally boosting to the immune system. So you have many options for application.

While you are making up your mind whether to rub it in or pop it down the hatch, or both, have a cup of tea. L-theanine, abundant in both black and green tea, is an amino acid vital to optimal immune system functioning but, even better, tea drinkers tend to have (according to Harvard studies) up to ten times more interferon (the virus-fighting agent) in their bloodstream.

Calendula and Salicylic Paste

Salicylic acid is abundant in the leaves and twigs of willow trees and in the foliage and tops of meadowsweet. Blitzing with calendula petals introduces the healing properties of vitamin A and skin rejuvenation phytochemicals. A few tablespoons of each are all you will need.

Method
Gather some meadowsweet or willow and mash up with a mortar and pestle or blitz in a blender with some coconut oil or green tea to produce a decent paste or pulp to apply. You only need a small amount and it will keep in the fridge for five days.

How best to use: the recommended treatment schedule is for a daily treatment over a ten-week period. Some verrucae resolve within a few months but return periodically, so the long treatment time is to ensure maximum damage to viral cells. You may wish to consult a chiropodist or naturopath to supplement or supervise treatment.

WARTS

Warts are a sign of a virus – the human papillomavirus (HPV) in fact – which causes the body to produce an excess of skin cells. The best way to tackle them is to attack the virus by boosting your immune system: diet, herbal teas and vitamin supplements will all help. Warts are easily spreadable around your own body and quite contagious. Scratching a wart and then, say, rubbing your neck or any skin surface can move the virus-filled cells around like seeds. In fact common warts are often referred to as seed warts. While most are largely painless, they are ugly and some can become uncomfortable and sore – especially on the fingers and thumbs chafed by gardening chores. Much like botrytis on tomato plants, they enter the system via cuts and nicks, often at moist sections of skin; so bare feet in work boots or bare hands in sweaty gloves provide the right incubation. Many warts will eventually resolve themselves, even without treatment, but it can take up to two years. That's two years of spreading potential – so, just like a weed, once spotted they're best eradicated.

Types of Warts

Common warts/'seed warts': rough, dome-shaped and typically found around the fingernails and backs of hands.

Plantar warts: 'seed type' found mainly on the sole of the foot and occasionally on toes.

Periungual warts: 'seed type' found mainly around fingernails and toenails.

Mosaic warts: a cluster of individual plantar-type warts on the body.

Filiform warts: long and narrow, predominantly facial warts.

Flat warts: flat formations slightly darker than your skin tone. Commonly located about arms, neck, face and forehead, but found at other locations too.

Genital warts: any growth on or proximate to the penis, anus or vulva/vagina needs medical attention: visit your GP or local STI clinic.

Garden treatments

Both wild and garden-grown euphorbias (along with other members of the spurge family) have been employed to burn off warts and other skin growths via dabs of their caustic milky sap. Similarly dandelion milk was once traditionally applied two to three times daily until the wart was eradicated. Celandine was utilised in this manner too. There are of course gentle garden options – a petal poultice of calendula (rich in vitamin A) can soften warts to enable pumicing off. Many over-the-counter treatments echo the ancient usage of willow sap treatment by employing salicylic acid in their ingredients. Extract your own salicylic acid by blending some willow tips and foliage in a little water or witch hazel extract and applying that twice daily until the wart shrinks away to nothing – helped along by some pumicing after each soak.

> ### Top tip
>
> As warts can be transferred in sloughed off skin cells, get a dedicated wart pumice stone and clean it thoroughly between uses. Some sudsy water with a few drops of thyme essential oil or a rinse with any spirit alcohol will sterilise it.

Kitchen support

The best way to tackle warts is to tackle the virus, so the immunity-boosting edibles on page 65 will help your system reboot and go on the attack. A lowered immune system or a fatigued person are more prone to warts – so some energy smoothies along with alternative or conventional treatments will treat the underlying cause too. The acidity of both lemon juice and apple cider vinegar topically applied will provide some gentle corrosion and cell altering that will force our immune system to 'pick up' the 'blip' and deal with it. The vitamin C content in the fruit juice is also beneficial for the recovery of skin after the wart has been eradicated, as well as contributing to the destruction of the virus causing the wart. You can also boost the mix with some pineapple juice and garlic or onion juice. Use in compresses, corn plasters or as direct drops.

Retinoid treatment: retinoid cream (derived from vitamin A) is often employed in dermatological clinics, beauty salons or via GP prescription. It can be quite effective at checking the growth of warts as vitamin A disrupts the warts' cellular development. It can be as easily sourced from capsule supplements as from expensive creams, or you could try a home-pressed pumpkin seed or apricot kernel oil. If home pressing puts you off, then a mortar and pestle can yield an A-rich seed paste. Of course there is always good old sunflower oil too (add some macerated calendula petals for an extra boost). Eating vitamin-A-rich foods will also boost immune function.

See also the echinacea and thyme tincture, page 70, for topical and internal applications.

WEIGHT GAIN

We all gain unwanted pounds from time to time, and it is OK to not want to keep them or complicate our health, but obsessing or yo-yo or crash dieting is not a great way to live. Fad diets can be health disasters down the line, so if you need to lose some weight or just tone up an extra notch before holidays then, apart from more exercise and eating fewer calories, there are some nutritional tricks you can employ to boost the success of your endeavours – and the garden can help too.

Garden treatments

Remember, the garden is a green gym! Mowing a lawn with a push mower for half an hour burns 243 calories in exertion – that is equivalent to the strenuous activity of chopping wood for a half hour. Turning a compost pile for approximately 15 minutes can burn in excess of 100 calories. Lifting a gallon watering can full of water in each hand is equivalent to 8-pound dumbbells. Raking has the potential to burn approximately 324 calories per hour, while more strenuous tilling or digging can burn approximately 404 calories per hour. A mix of activities will burn calories more effectively and work different muscle groups.

Simple gardening tasks can burn up those extra pounds without you noticing the effort or experiencing the stress of avoiding or missing the gym. The physicality of gardening not only benefits muscles, bones and organs but also releases endorphins, which help to alleviate stress and its side effects – including comfort eating and binge eating. A healthy portion of gardening will stimulate real appetite (learning the difference between hunger and boredom is key in weight management) and foster a good night's sleep (intrinsic to effective metabolism). Gardening provides more than aerobic exercise through the physicality associated with gardening as a pastime: it also provides isotonic and isometric exercise. This trinity of exercise modes increases strength, endurance and flexibility – so a real fitness boost and the knock-on boost to your sense of well-being, good mood and motivation to stick with healthy eating and regular exercise.

Kitchen support

Dieting can cause your body to think it's starving and so hold onto calories when you next eat. Eat less junk but more nutrition. So while you try to consume less, the 'dietary not diet' remedy contains some items you might want to consume more of.

DIETARY NOT DIET

- Enjoy a cup of *green tea* each day – it's packed with fat-burning phytochemical compounds known as catechins. One of those catechins, epigallocatechin gallate, is an antioxidant that protects the hormone norepinephrine. Norepinephrine, amongst other things, is the signal system to fat cells to instigate the breakdown of fat. More green tea means more norepinephrine telling those fat cells that you mean business.
- Eat foods that are rich in *zinc* – not just for the health

benefit of zinc in its own right but because zinc helps boost the activity of the hormone leptin which tells your brain when you should feel full and to stop eating. Leptin also regulates fat storage and increases energy expenditure. Zinc-rich foods include pumpkin seeds, spinach, nuts and beans. Zinc requires vitamin B6 for proper absorption.

- *Vitamin B6* will help zinc activate that hunger-killing leptin hormone but another of its roles is to assist in the conversion of glycogen (stored sugar) to glucose (fuel), so in burning stored calories we raise the energy potential of the body and diminish the need for more carbs to refuel our functions. B6 is in sunflower seeds, pistachio nuts, avocados, spinach and many common foods.

- *Calcium* is perhaps less known for its role in both energy metabolism and regulation of body composition. It doesn't have to be found in dairy – calcium is also in garden greens, so a salad or leafy veg option each day for lunch will result in a lower body mass index. To maximise calcium's potential you can lunch al fresco – that extra daylight (vitamin D) promotes calcium absorption.

- *Vitamin C* does wonderful things for the body beautiful and our health in general but in terms of weight management it is essential for the production of a compound called carnitine, which encourages the body to turn fat into fuel and not just store it. Beyond citrus fruits, try bell peppers and dark leafy greens.

WEIGHT LOSS

Weight loss can be an underlying health issue (adrenal, thyroid or liver disorder) and certainly any sudden drops in weight should always be investigated by a GP. It can be related to metabolism or indeed malabsorption in the digestive tract. It may be that you are eating less lately but are physically more active. It may be stress related (see page 237).

Garden treatments

Dandelion as salad herb or root coffee has the ability to stimulate the appetite. Gentian has phytoestrogens that help the body store more calories and it also helps the body to absorb food and sustenance much more efficiently – enabling bulk not burn. These are just two of many 'bitter herbs' (see page 99) that stimulate appetite.

Kitchen support

Protein will help. Not skipping carbs will help. Not bingeing but having healthier portions and good quality food is part of the solution. The spice fenugreek is used to prompt weight gain in some cultures where bigger women are traditionally prized. It contains properties similar to oestrogen that help the body hold on to calories – many thinner people have more muscle fibre which causes them to burn more energy, even while resting, so holding on to calories is vital. Fenugreek in fresh leaf form can be used as a pot herb – known also as methi: it is a staple of

Indian cooking. 'Kasoori Methi' is its dried form and a cooking herb. The seeds are used whole and ground to make spice. Either can be used as a tea, added to other herbal teas or simply used in cooking.

Kinda Aloo Ko Achar

My take on Nepalese fenugreek potato salad, but lightly pan-fried, for two.

Ingredients

- 6–7 salad potatoes
- ⅓ cup garden peas
- 2 tablespoons lemon juice
- 1 tablespoon honey
- 1 scallion or 2 tablespoons diced onion
- 1 green chilli
- ⅓ cup methi or substitute with coriander leaves
- 1 tablespoon butter
- 1 teaspoon turmeric
- 1 teaspoon fenugreek seeds
- Pinch of black pepper

Method

Boil the potatoes in salted water until cooked through. Add the peas near the end to just lightly cook. Strain and set aside to cool a little. Mix together the lemon juice and honey. Slice or dice the scallion. Slice or dice the chilli. Next, quarter or cut the potatoes into cubes – I like to keep the skin on but you can peel them if you prefer. Mix all the veg together. Add the honey and lemon and fold in the methi. Then, to a hot skillet or frying pan, add the butter, turmeric and fenugreek seeds – once the seeds brown add the potato mix and sizzle for a moment, enough to partially crisp the underneath. Turn out onto a plate, add a pinch of black pepper and enjoy.

WINTER VOMITING BUG/ NOROVIRUS

The winter vomiting bug is a name given to seasonal outbreaks of norovirus – the same agent for gastroenteritis (see page 230) and sundry digestive system upsets. It presents with stomach pain, cramping, diarrhoea (see page 95), nausea and vomiting (see page 204), with ancillary symptoms of elevated temperature, dehydration and fatigue (see page 123). It is highly contagious. Incubation is on average twelve to forty-eight hours, with the illness normally persisting for one to three days but it can, with younger children and older adults, extend for four to six days. Age can affect symptoms too, with diarrhoea more prevalent in adults and vomiting the main symptom in children.

Garden treatments

The phytochemicals in elderberries have the ability to disarm viruses, including norovirus. Many garden-grown antimicrobial herbs (oregano, rosemary, lavender, thyme) can also help to damage or destroy viral particles. Immunostimulants such as astragalus, andrographis and echinacea can build your white cell count up to army strength. Echinacea is renowned for fighting infections – it is full of an antibiotic phytochemical called echinacoside, capable of destroying or limiting a broad range of bacteria, fungi and protozoa, and also viruses. Echinacea not only agitates the immune system into creating more T cells (to fight off foreign bodies like viruses), it also boosts the ability of our macrophages to physically destroy and remove viral content from our system. Thyme is naturally bactericidal and fungicidal but it is also antiviral – its phytochemicals actively kill microbes and trigger the formation of more white blood cells. Oregano acts in a similar way. See also stomach upsets (page 230).

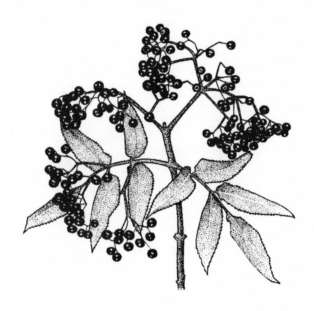

Elderberries

Kitchen support

Dehydration is an issue so drink plenty of fluids. Start by having a cup of tea – an amino acid vital to optimal immune system functioning known as L-theanine is abundant in both black and green tea. Green tea not only stimulates the liver to secrete interferon, but it contains many potent antioxidant compounds to neutralise free radicals that inhibit the healthy functioning of our immune system.

Coconut water is restorative and full of electrolytes to re-hydrate. Chamomile tea can settle the stomach and calm nerves. Try also rice water (the water you have boiled rice in), as it supplies some nourishment to the convalescing system and it also helps to constipate – meaning less diarrhoea. Apple cider vinegar is a natural detoxicant, which cleanses without depleting vital nutrients from the system. Vitamin B6, found in sunflower seeds, sesame seeds, pumpkin and squash seeds as well as nuts and raisins, supports immune function. One of the best approaches is to eat bland foods for a few days – avoid spices and condiments, sugar-loaded and processed foods.

B6 Flapjack

A sweet and filling treat for convalescent nutrition and immune-system support.

Ingredients

- 175g butter
- 175g honey
- 175g sugar
- 1 tablespoon apple juice
- 1 teaspoon lemon juice
- ½ cup raisins
- 2 tablespoons wheatgerm
- 2 tablespoons sunflower seeds
- 2 tablespoons sesame seeds
- 2 tablespoons flaked almonds
- 350g rolled oats

Method

Preheat the oven to 150°C/300°F/Gas Mark 2. In a saucepan, melt the butter, honey and sugar together with the juices to form a syrup, then turn off the heat and add all the dry ingredients – stir well together. Scoop the mix into a 9-inch (23cm) square baking tin lined with parchment paper. Place in the oven and bake for 35 minutes. Remove to a chopping board and allow to cool completely before cutting into squares.

INDEX OF PLANTS

INDEX OF AILMENTS

INDEX OF RECIPES

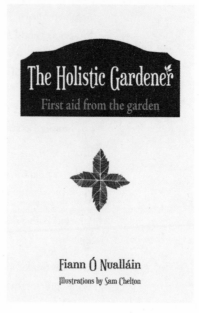

A handy guide to quick and effective natural first-aid treatments for commonly occurring accidents and complaints, derived from garden and kitchen sources.

From a thorn prick to heatstroke, from chapped hands to hay fever, from pesticide poisoning to wasp stings: all of these can be treated on site with what you grow. The plant beside you as you work or relax in the garden can be the answer to the hive, ache or watery eye.

Written by a professional gardener with a lifetime's experience of accidents that can happen in the garden, all the information you need on first response, the essential plants and homemade remedy preparation is combined in this book.

www.mercierpress.ie

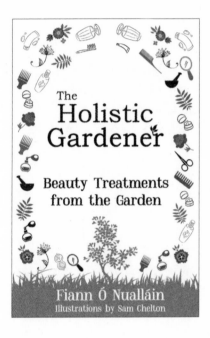

Even the smallest garden or container can be a rich source of cosmetic plants and healing herbs to boost the body beautiful. This book brings together everything you need to know about feeling great, looking amazing and taking control of your beauty regime using all-natural products. It explores not just which plants whiten teeth, strengthen nails, alleviate dandruff or build collagen, but also which treatments are as effective as, or sometimes better than, shop-bought products.

Containing step-by-step recipes for creams, balms, tonics and product substitutes, and targeted nutritional advice to nourish every part of your body and treat common beauty complaints, this is a DIY beauty bible, showing you how to look good and feel great, naturally.

www.mercierpress.ie